SUCCESS!

Phlebotomy

A Q&A Exam Review

Seventh Edition

Kathleen Becan-McBride, EdD, MLS(ASCP)[CM]
Director, Community and Educational Outreach
Coordinator, Texas–Mexico Border Health Services
Medical School Professor in the Department of Family and Community Medicine
The University of Texas Health Science Center at Houston
Texas Medical Center, Houston, Texas
Assistant Director for Academic Partnerships, Greater Houston AHEC

Diana Garza, EdD, MLS(ASCP)[CM]
Medical Writer/Editor
Health Care Consultant
Houston, Texas

Pearson
Boston Columbus Indianapolis New York San Francisco Upper Saddle River
Amsterdam Cape Town Dubai London Madrid Milan Munich Paris Montreal
Delhi Mexico City São Paulo Sydney Hong Kong Seoul Singapore Taipei

Library of Congress Cataloging-in-Publication Data

Becan-McBride, Kathleen,
Success! in phlebotomy : a Q&A exam review / Kathleen Becan-McBride, Diana Garza. — 7th ed.
p. ; cm.
Rev. ed. of: Prentice Hall's Q & A for phlebotomy / Kathleen Becan-McBride, Diana Garza. 6th ed. c2006.
Includes index.
ISBN-13: 978-0-13-510100-1
ISBN-10: 0-13-510100-X
1. Phlebotomy—Examinations, questions, etc. I. Garza, Diana. II. Becan-McBride, Kathleen, 1949- Prentice Hall's Q & A for phlebotomy. III. Title.
[DNLM: 1. Phlebotomy—Examination Questions. QY 18.2 B388s 2010]
RB45.15.G37 2010 Suppl.
616.07'561076—dc22

2010000431

Publisher: Julie Levin Alexander
Editor-in-Chief: Mark Cohen
Development Editor: Melissa Kerian
Assistant Editor: Nicole Ragonese
Media Editor: Amy Peltier
Media Project Manager: Lorena Cerisano
Executive Marketing Manager: Katrin Beacom
Marketing Assistant: Judy Noh
Production Manager: Fran Russello
Composition/Full-Service Project Management: Chitra Ganesan/GGS Higher Education Resources, A division of PreMedia Global Inc.
Printer/Binder: Hamilton Printing Co.
Cover printer: Lehigh-Phoenix

Pearson Education LTD., London
Pearson Education Singapore, Pte. Ltd
Pearson Education, Canada, Inc.
Pearson Education–Japan
Pearson Education Australia PTY Limited
Pearson Education North Asia, Ltd. , Hong Kong
Pearson Educación de Mexico, S.A. de C.V.
Pearson Education Malaysia, Pte. Ltd.
Pearson Education, Upper Saddle River, New Jersey

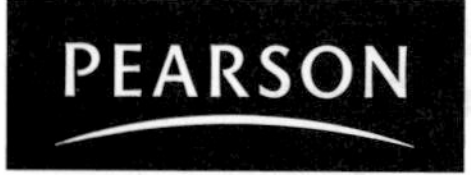

www.pearsonhighered.com

10 9 8 7 6 5 4 3

ISBN-(13): 978-0-13-510100-1
ISBN-(10): 0-13-510100-X

To my husband, Mark; my sons, Patrick and Jonathan and daughter-in-law, Danielle; my grandson, Finnaveir; my granddaughter, Madeleine; my parents; my sister; and my mother-in-law for their support and devotion.

—Kathleen Becan-McBride

To my husband, Peter McLaughlin; my children, Lauren, Kaitlin, and Kevin; and my parents for their affection, patience, and constant support.

—Diana Garza

Contents

Preface

The number of clinical laboratory techniques, automated instruments, and analyses continues to escalate, increasing the demand for proper collection of patient laboratory specimens. Since the majority of laboratory errors occur in the preanalytical phase, it is essential that health care students and practitioners who are responsible for blood and other specimen collections (i.e., phlebotomists, medical laboratory technologists and technicians, nurses, respiratory therapists, and others) have an in-depth knowledge of their professional responsibilities. The responsibilities of the blood collector continue to rise and encompass additional patient care and clinical activities. National board certification in phlebotomy is required by many health care institutions, clinics, and physicians' offices as a result of federal, safety, and quality assurance requirements. The rationale for phlebotomy certification and state licensure is gaining momentum nationally and internationally. Because of these regulations and laws to ensure high-quality patient care, continuing education (CE) in phlebotomy safety and quality assurance has become paramount.

These important events in the responsibilities of blood collection have served to shape the seventh edition of ***SUCCESS! in Phlebotomy.*** It has been designed to act as a study companion for those who are (1) preparing for international, national or state board certification/licensure examinations and/or (2) pursuing self-assessment in blood collection.

SUCCESS! in Phlebotomy, **Seventh Edition,** includes multiple-choice questions as a means to the overall review of blood collection, handling, and transportation. The chapters in this book are sequenced to match the order of those in the ***Phlebotomy Handbook: Blood Collection Essentials,*** **Eighth Edition.** The question-and-answer contents are divided into the following major sections:

- SECTION I: Overview and Safety Procedures—provides questions and answers related to: (1) the roles and functions of phlebotomists in the health care industry, (2) safety and infection control in the workplace, and (3) basics of anatomy and physiology with an emphasis on the circulatory system.
- SECTION II: Phlebotomy Equipment and Procedures—provides questions and answers related to: (1) the latest phlebotomy equipment and supplies, (2) techniques used in phlebotomy, (3) documentation and transportation procedures needed for safe handling of biohazardous specimens, and (4) complications that may occur during the procedures.
- SECTION III: Point-of-Care Testing and Special Procedures—provides questions and answers related to: (1) pediatric phlebotomy procedures, (2) arterial and IV collections, and (3) special considerations for the older, homebound, and long-term-care patients.

Each chapter includes chapter objectives as a guide. After the reader learns the essential topics in the ***Phlebotomy Handbook: Blood Specimen Collection from Basic to Advanced,*** **Eighth Edition,** he or she can review them through the questions and answers presented in this book. Alternatively, this book may stand alone as a review book because it contains explanatory answers as well. All of these answers have references to pages in the ***Phlebotomy Handbook: Blood Specimen Collection from Basic to Advanced,*** **Eighth Edition,** so that the reader can obtain additional information on the question topic. This review book incorporates updated illustrations of blood collection equipment and techniques as bases for questions to help sharpen phlebotomy skills. A corresponding website, *www.myhealthprofessionskit.com*, features additional practice and resources.

Using this book will assist the reader in identifying areas of relative strength and weakness in the command of phlebotomy skills and responsibilities. After reviewing the multiple-choice questions and answers, the reader can practice taking the simulated examination provided on the accompanying website.

SUCCESS! in Phlebotomy, **Seventh Edition,** ***Phlebotomy Handbook: Blood Specimen Collection from Basic to Advanced,*** **Eighth Edition,** and the ***Instructor's Resource Manual*** to accompany the ***Phlebotomy Handbook***

are major *national* and *international* references for health care providers' educational programs, hospitals, physicians' offices, clinics, national examination boards, and legal issues in blood collection.

References

Garza, D., & Becan-McBride, K. (2010). *Phlebotomy Handbook: Blood Specimen Collection from Basic to Advanced* (8th ed.). Upper Saddle River, NJ: Pearson.

Kathleen Becan-McBride
Diana Garza

Reviewers

Rhonda Anderson, PBT (ASCP)^{CM}
Greenville Technical College
Greenville, South Carolina

Carry Deatley, AAS, BA, MBA
Southern State Community College
Hillsboro, Ohio

Penny Ewing, BS, CMA (AAMA)
Gaston College
Dallas, North Carolina

Judy Ward, CMA (AAMA), PBT (ASCP), NREMT-P
Ivy Tech Community College
Indianapolis, Indiana

Introduction

SUCCESS!

ABOUT THE SUCCESS! SERIES

SUCCESS! is a complete exam preparation system that combines relevant exam-style questions with outline-style content review and interactive technology.

This format provides you with the best preparation for your exam!

- Build your experience and exam confidence!
- Practice with realistic exam-style questions.
- Enhance your review with state-of-the-art technology that offers more practice.

The **SUCCESS!** program is a proven method for increasing pass rates in many health professions from EMS to nursing. We invite you to use our exam preparation system and HAVE SUCCESS!

Pearson's complete **SUCCESS!** system includes review for the following areas:

Medical laboratory science	Dental hygiene
Dental assisting	Emergency medical services
Health information management	Nursing assisting

Home health aid	Pharmacy technician
Massage therapy	Phlebotomy
Medical assisting	Surgical technology

Visit *www.pearsonhighered.com/health* professions for more information on these or other Pearson Health titles.

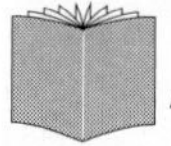

ABOUT SUCCESS! IN PHLEBOTOMY

Part of the **SUCCESS!** Series, ***SUCCESS! in Phlebotomy,*** **Seventh Edition,** offers you a comprehensive approach to phlebotomy review. The question-and-answer review in the book and the practice exam on the corresponding website provide the practice needed for SUCCESS! on the ASCP, and NPA certification exams and other certification and state licensure exams.

In the Book

Chapter Objectives
Each chapter opens with objectives that allow you to preview the topics discussed. At a glance you will be able to identify the information and skills that you are responsible for knowing.

Realistic Exam-Style Questions
This review book contains 850 exam-style multiple-choice questions organized by topic area. Working through these questions will help you assess your strengths and weaknesses in each topic of study. These questions have been written at three different levels that consist of:

- *Recall*—the ability to recall previously memorized knowledge, skills, and facts
- *Applications*—the ability to apply recalled knowledge in verbal and written skills
- *Problem solving*—the ability to apply recalled knowledge in solving a problem or case situation

Answers and Rationales
For each question in the book, the answer is provided with feedback allowing you to fully comprehend the answer.

References
Enhance your review by referencing ***Phlebotomy Handbook: Blood Specimen Collection from Basic to Advanced,*** **Eighth Edition,** by Diana Garza and Kathleen Becan-McBride as you practice with ***SUCCESS! in Phlebotomy,*** **Seventh Edition.** Answers to all questions contained in ***SUCCESS! in Phlebotomy,*** **Seventh Edition,** also include references to the best-selling title ***Phlebotomy Handbook: Blood Specimen Collection from Basic to Advanced,*** **Eighth Edition,** allowing you to easily find more information and in-depth information on a specific topic area.

On the Website

Visit *www.myhealthprofessionskit.com* for additional practice questions, an audio glossary, and links to related resources. Designed to enhance your review, you will want to bookmark this site as you continue on your path to SUCCESS!

CERTIFICATION

Each of at least six organizations currently has certification tests in phlebotomy. If you intend to apply for one or more of the certification examinations, determine which particular phlebotomy certification examinations are better known and/or accepted in your local community and state. Sometimes health care organizations have preferences for specific certifications and will adjust salaries accordingly. Likewise, local community colleges, universities, and health care institutions can also provide recommendations about which certification examination to take.

Also, some states are pursuing licensing of phlebotomists, which is required if you intend to work in that state. As an example, California requires state licensure for phlebotomists and certain training and experience requirements similar to the national board requirements. Since some states have credentialing or CE requirements for phlebotomists, it is important to know which organizations are approved by state health departments to provide the examination or CE programs.

The organizations listed next have an interest in promoting and improving the practice of phlebotomy. They differ slightly in their membership requirements, fees, member benefits, CE courses, and/or to the degree that they offer certification specifically for phlebotomists.

NONPROFIT ORGANIZATIONS

The National Phlebotomy Association (NPA)
1901 Brightseat Road
Landover, MD 20785
(301) 386-4200
(301) 386-4203 (fax)
www.nationalphlebotomy.org

NPA was established in 1978 to recognize the phlebotomist as a distinctive and identifiable part of the health care team. NPA has established professional standards, a code of ethics, educational opportunities, and an annual certification examination resulting in a CPT (NPA). NPA has trained and certified approximately 15,000 phlebotomists in all 50 states and abroad and has accredited 75 teaching programs. Accredited programs must include the following topic areas: historical perspective, medical terminology, anatomy and physiology, communication, phlebotomy practical, cardiopulmonary resuscitation (CPR), stress management, phlebotomy techniques, human relations, legal aspects, infection control, and drug awareness.

American Medical Technologists (AMT)
10700 West Higgins Road, Suite 150
Rosemont, IL 60018
(847) 823-5169 or (800) 275-1268
(847) 823-0458 (fax)
www.amt1.com

AMT offers a certification examination for registered phlebotomy technician (RPT).

National Accrediting Agency for Clinical Laboratory Sciences (NAACLS)
8410 West Bryn Mawr Avenue, Suite 670
Chicago, IL 60631
(773) 714-8880
(773) 714-8886 (fax)
www.naacls.org

NAACLS accredits educational programs in clinical laboratory sciences including phlebotomy. No certification examinations are provided.

The American Society for Clinical Pathology (ASCP)
Board of Certification
33 W. Monroe Street, Suite 1600
Chicago, IL 60603
(312) 541-4999; (800) 267-2727
www.ascp.org

ASCP offers many levels of certification, through the Board of Certification Registry, including a Phlebotomy Technician Examination, PBT (ASCP), and an international certification examination for PBTs. It also provides educational programs, teleconferences, webinars, and workshops; phlebotomy scholarships; and online CE for phlebotomists. The certification exam covers the entry-level skills of a phlebotomist and uses taxonomy levels that assess recall (recognize facts), interpretive skills (use knowledge to interpret numeric data), and problem-solving skills (use applications of specific information to solve problems). Over 15,000 phlebotomists have been certified by ASCP since 1989.

American Society of Phlebotomy Technicians (ASPT)
P.O. Box 1831
Hickory, NC 28603
(828) 294-0078
(828) 327-2969 (fax)
www.aspt.org

ASPT offers a certification examination that results in a CPT (ASPT) certification. It also offers certification examinations for point-of-care technician, EKG technician, drug collection specialist, paramedical insurance examiner, and patient care technician.

COMMERCIAL ORGANIZATIONS

National Healthcareer Association (NHA)
National Headquarters
7 Ridgedale Avenue, Suite 203
Cedar Knolls, NJ 07927
(973) 605-1881 or (800) 499-9092
(973) 644-4797 (fax)
www.nha2000.com

Established in 1989, NHA was formed to create a network for health care professionals. NHA offers a certification examination for phlebotomists, CPT.

National Center for Competency Testing (NCCT/MMCI)
7007 College Blvd, Suite 705
Overland Park, KS 66211
(800) 875-4404
(913) 498-1243 (fax)
www.ncctinc.com

NCCT provides certification and CE for phlebotomy technicians and instructors.

American Certification Agency (ACA)
P.O. Box 58
Osceola, IN 46561
(574) 277-4538
(574) 277-4624 (fax)
www.acacert.com

ACA provides certification examinations for phlebotomy technicians and instructors.

As mentioned earlier, some states require that laboratory personnel be licensed before working in the field. State licensing may require an additional test, or the state may utilize one of the certification examinations provided by a professional organization such as those listed earlier. To maintain licensing and/or certification credentials, phlebotomists must also participate in **CE** activities. In addition, some health care organizations prefer specific certifications over others, so it may be beneficial to check with local employers and state health departments prior planning for a certification examination.

STUDY TIPS

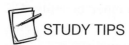

Review Materials

Know how the test is set up, the test-day procedures, and how much time you have. Choose review materials that contain the information you need to study. Save time by making sure that you aren't studying anything you don't need to. Before the exam, the best study preparation would be to use this Question & Answer Review to identify your strengths and weaknesses. The references at the end of each rationale will direct you to additional resources for more in-depth study.

Set a Study Schedule

Use your time-management skills to set a schedule that will help you feel as prepared as you can be. Consider all the relevant factors—the materials you need to study; how many months, weeks, or days until the test date; and how much time you can study each day. If you establish your schedule ahead of time and write it in your date book, you will be much more likely to follow it. It is helpful to include in your date book a list of the items that you plan on studying each day and the amount of time allotted to studying those items each day. Then after studying for that day, you can check that day's list off and feel confident that you know that section of phlebotomy material. This strategy keeps you from procrastinating one more day from studying for the upcoming exam!

Take Practice Tests

Practice as much as possible, using the questions in this book and on the web. These questions were designed to follow the format of questions that appear on the exam you will take, so the more you practice with these questions, the better prepared you will be on test day. Repetition in answering the phlebotomy questions correctly is the key to learning the phlebotomy materials and preparing effectively for the actual exam.

The practice tests on the website will give you a chance to experience the exam before you actually have to take it and will also let you know how you're doing and where you need to improve. For best results, we recommend you take a practice test 2–3 weeks before you are scheduled to take the actual exam. Spend the next weeks targeting those areas in which you performed poorly by reviewing questions in those areas.

Practice under test-like conditions—in a quiet room, with no books or notes to help you, and with a clock telling you when to quit. Try to come as close as you can to duplicating the actual test situation.

TAKING THE EXAMINATION

Prepare Physically

When taking the exam, you need to work efficiently under time pressure. If your body is tired or under stress, you might not think as clearly or perform as well as you usually do. If you can, avoid staying up all night. Get enough sleep so that you can wake up rested and alert.

Eating right is also important. The best advice is to eat a light, well-balanced meal before a test. When time is short, grab a quick-energy snack such as a banana, orange juice, or a granola bar.

The Examination Site

The examination site is usually selected at the time of registration; locate it before the required examination time. One suggestion is to find the site and parking facilities the day before the test. Also find out how much parking will cost so that sufficient money can be taken along on the examination day.

Allow plenty of time for travel to the site in case of unexpected mishaps such as traffic snarls. During travel, think positive thoughts (e.g., My preparation for the exam was thorough, so I'll be able to answer the questions easily). Maintain a confident attitude to prevent unnecessary stress. Also, deep breathing is an excellent stress reducer, especially in preparation for taking the major exam! Prior to taking the exam, breathe by tucking in your stomach and feel the air as it expands your lungs. Hold your breath for four counts and then exhale for a total count of four. This breathing technique has a calming effect and will assist you in focusing on answering each exam question.

Materials

Be sure to take all required identification materials (usually a photo ID), registration forms, and any other items required by the testing organization or center. Read information and instructions supplied by the testing organizations thoroughly to make sure that you have all the necessary materials (e.g., a nonprogrammable calculator) before the day of the exam. Do not carry textbooks or notes into the testing area. Scratch paper is often provided if needed. Remember, you will *not* be allowed to take the test if you forget any of the required forms or identification. And don't be surprised if you are fingerprinted and/or photographed when you enter the examination room. It is a standard procedure at some testing centers to assure identity each time you enter and return to the room.

Read Test Directions

Read the examination directions thoroughly! Because some board examinations have different test sections with different question formats, it is important to be aware of changes in directions. Read each set of directions completely before starting a new section of questions.

Computerized Exams

To ensure that you are comfortable with the computer test format, be sure to practice on the computer using the CD-ROM that is included in the back of this book.

Since certification exam requirements vary, determine before taking a computerized exam whether you can change your answer after you strike a key for a particular answer. Checking your answers is an very important part of taking a major certification exam. Thus, do not enter an answer on a computerized exam unless you (1) have the option to change it as you are checking your answers or (2) are absolutely certain that your answer is correct when you first enter it.

During the exam, check the computer screen after an answer is entered to verify that the answer appears as it was entered. If you feel fatigued, close your eyes, take a few deep breaths, and stretch your arms and shoulders; then resume the examination. If you need assistance, check to see if there is a "HELP" function or contact the testing proctor.

Pencil and Paper Exams

Machine-scored tests require that you use a pencil to fill in a small box on a computerized answer sheet. Use the right pencil (usually a No. 2), and mark your answers in the correct space. Neatness counts on these tests, because the computer can misread stray pencil marks or partially erased answers. Periodically, check the answer number against the question number to make sure they match. One question skipped can cause every answer following it to be marked incorrectly.

Selecting the Right Answer

Keep in mind that only one answer is correct. First read the stem of the question with *each* possible choice provided and eliminate choices that are obviously incorrect. Be cautious about choosing the first answer that *might* be correct; all possibilities should be considered before the final choice is made; the best answer should be selected. If a question is complicated, try to break it down into small sections that are easy to understand. Pay special attention to qualifiers such as *only, except,* etc. For example, negative words in a question can confuse your understanding of what the question asks ("Which of the following is *not* . . .?").

Intelligent Guessing

If you don't know the answer, eliminate those answers that you know or suspect are wrong. Your goal is to narrow down your choices. Here are some questions to ask yourself:

- Is the choice accurate in its own terms? If there's an error in the choice, for example, a term that is incorrectly defined—the answer is wrong.
- Is the choice relevant? An answer may be accurate, but it may not relate to the essence of the question. Choose the answer that is the most logical answer to you.
- Are there any distractors, such as *always, never, all, none,* or *every?* Qualifiers make it easy to find an exception that makes a choice incorrect.
- Is one possible answer longer than the others? Frequently, the longest answer when others are much shorter is the correct answer.
- Mark answers you are not sure of, and go back to them at the end of the test.

Ask yourself whether you would make the same guesses again. Chances are that you will leave your answers alone, but you may notice something that will make you change your mind—a qualifier that affects meaning or a remembered fact that will enable you to answer the question without guessing.

Watch the Clock

Keep track of how much time is left and how you are progressing. Wear a watch or bring a small clock with you to the test room since you may not be able to take your cell phone into the testing area. A wall clock may be broken, or there may be no clock at all.

Some students are so concerned about time that they rush through the exam and have time left over. In such situations, it's easy to leave early. The best approach, however, is to take your time. Stay until the end so that you can check your answers or, if the test is computerized, make sure you know how to "End" the test. Some exams provide a preliminary "Pass or Fail" result at the test site.

KEYS TO SUCCESS!

- Study, review, and practice.
- Keep a positive, confident attitude.
- Follow all directions on the examination.
- Do your best.

Good luck!

You are encouraged to visit http://www.pearsonhighered.com/success for an additional practice exam and additional tips on studying, test-taking, and other keys to success. At this stage of your education and career you will find these tips helpful.

Some of the study and test-taking tips were adapted from Keys to Effective Learning, Second Edition, *by Carol Carter, Joyce Bishop, and Sarah Lyman Kravits.*

CHAPTER

1 Phlebotomy Practice and Quality Essentials

chapter objectives

Upon completion of Chapter 1, the learner is responsible for the following:

1. Define phlebotomy and identify health professionals who perform phlebotomy procedures.
2. Identify the importance of phlebotomy procedures to the overall care of the patient.
3. List professional competencies for phlebotomists and key elements of a performance assessment.
4. List members of a health care team who interact with phlebotomists.
5. Describe the roles of clinical laboratory personnel and common laboratory departments/sections.
6. Describe health care settings in which phlebotomy services are routinely performed.
7. Explain components of professionalism and desired character traits for phlebotomists.
8. Describe coping skills that are used for stress in the workplace.

9. List the basic tools used in quality improvement activities and give examples of how a phlebotomist can participate in quality improvement activities.
10. Define the difference between quality improvement and quality control.

DIRECTIONS Each of the questions or incomplete statements below is followed by four suggested answers or completions. Select one answer that is best in each case.

1. Most health care organizations fit into which of the following major categories of health care?
   A. specialty hospitals or clinics
   B. hospital or ambulatory care
   C. hospital or school based
   D. surgical or ambulatory centers

2. Job duties of phlebotomists can include which of the following?
   A. technical duties
   B. clinical duties only
   C. clinical, technical, and clerical duties
   D. technical and interpretive duties

3. Certification can provide advantages to phlebotomists in which of the following ways?
   A. automatic bonuses
   B. job opportunities, advancement, and portability
   C. improves accrued vacation time
   D. assures continuing education

4. The American Society for Clinical Pathology (ASCP) and the National Phlebotomy Association (NPA) are examples of what type of organization?
   A. licensing
   B. quality control
   C. certification
   D. accreditation

5. The health care department that uses radioactive isotopes or tracers in the diagnosis and treatment of patients and in the study of the disease process is the:
   A. clinical laboratory
   B. occupational therapy
   C. neurology
   D. nuclear medicine

6. Which of the following medical departments is associated with diagnostic and treatment procedures for bone and joint disorders and diseases?
   A. ophthalmology
   B. otolaryngology
   C. dermatology
   D. orthopedics

7. Which of the following departments deals with the general diagnosis and treatment of patients for problems of one or more internal organs?
   A. proctology
   B. anesthesiology
   C. internal medicine
   D. oncology

8. Which of the following sections is not a part of the clinical laboratory?
   A. radiology
   B. chemistry
   C. microbiology
   D. hematology

9. Which of the following departments dispenses medications?
   A. clinical laboratory
   B. pulmonary
   C. pharmacy
   D. radiology

10. What type of diploma is required to enter most phlebotomy training programs?
    A. high school or equivalent
    B. associate degree
    C. bachelor's degree
    D. master's degree

11. Which of the following departments deals with health care for children?
    A. pharmacy
    B. clinical laboratory
    C. radiology
    D. pediatrics

12. A primary consultant on the timing for collecting blood for drug levels is found in which of the following departments?
    A. pharmacy
    B. nutrition and dietetics
    C. occupational therapy
    D. clinical hematology

13. Biopsy tissue specimens are evaluated in which department?
    A. pulmonary
    B. urology
    C. clinical laboratory
    D. anatomic or surgical pathology

14. The attributes of good judgment, respecting patients' rights, and not harming anyone intentionally are examples of which of the following?
    A. ethical standards
    B. confidentiality statements
    C. competency statements
    D. rules of practice

15. A medical doctor who usually has extensive education in the study and diagnosis of diseases through the use of laboratory test results is sometimes referred to as a:
    A. medical laboratory technician (MLT)
    B. medical technologist
    C. clinical laboratory scientist (CLS)
    D. pathologist

16. Which of the following departments deals with disorders affecting the organs and tissues that produce hormones?
    A. neurology
    B. otolaryngology
    C. endocrinology
    D. nephrology

17. Which of the following character traits is vitally important to phlebotomists?
    A. personal integrity and veracity
    B. quickness and speed writing
    C. making rapid decisions
    D. having strong mathematical skills

18. Which of the following departments is involved in the diagnosis and treatment of malignant tumors?
    A. oncology
    B. rheumatology
    C. geriatrics
    D. proctology

19. Phlebotomists must always work with which of the following?
    A. personnel from the federal government
    B. only the laboratory personnel
    C. other members of the health care team
    D. assigned physicians in the hospital

20. The study of gastroenterology refers to the:
    A. nervous system
    B. ears, nose, and throat
    C. esophagus, stomach, and intestines
    D. organs and tissues that produce hormones

21. Mrs. J. Hamm, a patient who had blood tests requested from the nephrology department, probably has a disorder related to the:
    A. nervous system
    B. lungs
    C. kidneys
    D. immune system

22. Collecting a blood specimen from a patient's arm is an example of which phase of the laboratory workflow pathway?
    A. postanalytical
    B. analytical
    C. preanalytical
    D. maintenance

23. Most hospital laboratory departments have which of the following?
    A. radiotherapy department
    B. emergency rooms
    C. anatomical or surgical pathology and clinical pathology
    D. pharmacy testing

24. Ambulatory care refers to health care services provided to:
    A. inpatients
    B. outpatients
    C. patients in acute care hospitals
    D. patients in long-term care hospitals

25. Which of the following is *not* an important purpose of laboratory analyses for a health assessment of an individual?
    A. monitoring of the patient's health status
    B. developing a community needs assessment
    C. diagnostic testing on the patient
    D. therapeutic assessment to develop the appropriate treatment

26. For a certified phlebotomist, which of the following is an example of a professional competency?
    A. performs microscopic analysis of blood smears
    B. participates in the development of new laboratory testing instrumentation
    C. performs tests and records immunologic laboratory procedural results
    D. selects appropriate quality control procedures

27. Phlebotomists are primarily responsible for what phase of laboratory testing?
    A. preassessment
    B. preanalytical
    C. analytical
    D. postanalytical

28. The Centers for Medicare & Medicaid Services (CMS) regulates all clinical laboratories through which of the following?
    A. Clinical Laboratory Improvement Amendments of 1988 (CLIA '88)
    B. American Association of Blood Banks (AABB)
    C. Medicaid
    D. Medicare

29. Reporting final clinical laboratory test results is an example of which of the following?
    A. postanalytical
    B. analytical
    C. preanalytical
    D. maintenance

30. Eating a well-balanced diet, getting enough rest, and exercising can contribute to:
    A. cardiovascular disease
    B. stress reduction and a positive outlook
    C. mental conflicts among coworkers
    D. reduced performance at work

31. What is a phlebotomist required to do if she has long hair (several inches past her shoulders) and is working in a hospital laboratory as a phlebotomist?
    A. cut her hair to shoulder length
    B. cut her hair to be at the top of her neck
    C. pull/tie it back so that it is securely out of the way
    D. wear a cap to keep it away from her face

32. The clinical laboratory supervisor requested that Ms. Douglas, a phlebotomist, go quickly to the otolaryngology department to pick up a laboratory specimen belonging to Ms. Gonzales. The phlebotomist had to go to the department that provides treatment of the:
    A. eye
    B. ear, nose, and throat
    C. bones and joints
    D. skin

33. One type of shoe that is *not* recommended in a phlebotomist's dress code is:
    A. shoes that are clean and polished
    B. shoes that are quiet when walking
    C. sandals
    D. lace-up shoes

34. Six Sigma refers to which of the following?
    A. appropriateness of clinical care
    B. method of reducing variations to improve quality
    C. technical aspects of care
    D. interpersonal aspects of care

35. If the phlebotomist collects blood in the neonatology department, what type of patient is he or she performing blood collections on?
    A. hours to a few days old
    B. 3–5 years old
    C. 1–3 years old
    D. pregnant patients

36. Which of the following is a term used for a health care worker with a 2-year degree who has specimen collection duties and may perform designated tests and procedures?
    A. occupational therapist (OT)
    B. medical laboratory technician (MLT)
    C. clinical laboratory scientist (CLS)
    D. physical therapist (PT)

37. For CLIA '88 regulatory categories, which of the following is designated in the waived tests category?
    A. bone marrow evaluation
    B. urine culture
    C. urinalysis
    D. cytogenetics

38. The four categories that frame the concept of professionalism are:
    A. punctuality, attendance, respect, cleanliness
    B. respect, service, support, growth
    C. happiness, honesty, punctuality, commitment
    D. certification, licensure, accreditation, continuing education

39. One example of productivity measures for phlebotomy services is:
    A. patient waiting time
    B. hand hygiene
    C. courtesy
    D. gowning and gloving

40. In a health care setting, the internal customers do not include:
    A. physicians and medical students
    B. patients
    C. nurses and other allied health workers
    D. special interest groups

41. Which one of the following is an example of a quality control function?
    A. measuring the patient waiting times
    B. checking the temperature of a specimen refrigerator
    C. completing a customer satisfaction survey
    D. monitoring turn-around times for lab results

42. Which of the following departments in health care facilities has the specific responsibilities for the diagnosis and treatment of the elderly population ?
    A. geriatrics
    B. internal medicine
    C. psychiatry/neurology
    D. proctology

43. Which of the following patient specimens would most likely be taken to anatomic pathology?
    A. synovial fluid
    B. breast biopsy
    C. cerebrospinal fluid
    D. sputum

44. According to the CLIA '88, the cytogenetics analysis and electrophoresis tests are considered to be:
    A. waived
    B. extremely high-complexity
    C. high-complexity
    D. moderate-complexity

45. The PDCA cycle represents which of the following?
    A. quality model for performing venipunctures
    B. strategy to plan, do, check, and act
    C. plan, design, carry-out, assess
    D. Ten-step process for laboratory testing

46. Cause-and-effect diagrams can be used in quality improvement methodologies and are designed to:
    A. stimulate creative ideas
    B. break out components into a flowchart
    C. make bar charts that show the frequency of problems
    D. identify interactions among people, methods, equipment, and supplies

47. Pareto charts can be used in quality improvement methodologies and are designed to:
    A. make bar charts that show the frequency of problems
    B. stimulate creative ideas
    C. identify interactions among people, methods, equipment, and supplies
    D. break out components into a flowchart

48. Flowcharts can be used in quality improvement methodologies and are designed to:
    A. break out components into a diagram to understand a process
    B. make bar charts that show the frequency of problems
    C. stimulate creative ideas
    D. identify interactions among people, methods, equipment, and supplies

49. Quality improvement efforts for specimen collection frequently involve all but which one?
    A. phlebotomist's technique
    B. recollection rates
    C. frequency of hematomas
    D. negative drug reactions

50. An example of an outcomes assessment for a phlebotomy service's quality improvement plan can include:
    A. hematoma formation—number and size
    B. the presence of a pathologist 24 hours per day
    C. the number of fire extinguishers available
    D. organizational chart

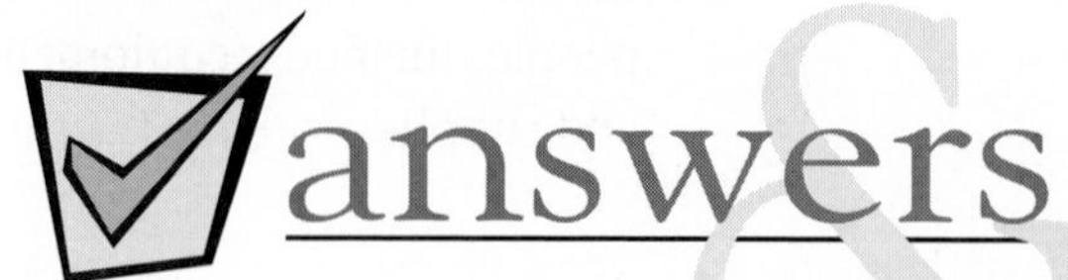

answers & rationales

1.

B. Most health care organizations in the United States fit into two major categories: hospital (inpatient) or ambulatory (outpatient) care. (p. 3)

2.

C. Phlebotomists are often expected to perform clinical, technical, and clerical duties. (p. 16)

3.

B. Certification provides phlebotomists with career advantages through increased job opportunities, advancement opportunities, and portability (the ability to carry the certification from state to state). (p. 11)

4.

C. ASCP and NPA are examples of national nonprofit agencies that provide certification examinations for phlebotomists. (pp. 12–13)

5.

D. The nuclear medicine department uses radioactive isotopes or tracers in the diagnosis and treatment of patients and in the study of the disease process. (p. 5)

6.

D. The orthopedics department performs diagnostic and treatment procedures for bone and joint disorders and diseases. (p. 6)

7.

C. Internal medicine is the department involved in the general diagnosis and treatment of patients for problems of one or more internal organs. (p. 5)

8.

A. The radiology department is not a part of the clinical laboratory. (pp. 5, 8)

9.

C. The pharmacy dispenses medications ordered by physicians. Pharmacists collaborate with phlebotomists when monitoring drug levels. (p. 6)

10.

A. A high school diploma or its equivalent is most often required to enter a phlebotomy training program. (p. 11)

11.

D. Pediatric departments deal with diagnoses of and therapy for children. (p. 5)

12.

A. The pharmacy department dispenses medications ordered by the physician and collaborates with the health care team on drug therapies. Typically, the clinical chemistry section works closely with the pharmacy department on establishing correct timing for drug levels. (p. 6)

13.

D. Surgical biopsy specimens are analyzed in the anatomic or surgical pathology department. (p. 7)

14.

A. These are examples of ethical standards of performance that are common to most professional organizations in the health care industry. (p. 17)

15.

D. A pathologist is a physician who has extensive training in pathology, which is the study and diagnosis of diseases through the use of laboratory test results. (p. 11)

16.

C. The endocrinology department deals with disorders affecting organs and tissues that produce hormones. (p. 4)

17.

A. While quickness, making fast decisions, and speed writing can be helpful, they are not important traits when dealing with patients. It is more important to take time to perform duties carefully and thoroughly. Personal integrity and veracity involve telling the truth and doing things right when no one is looking. These traits are vitally important for a phlebotomist. (p. 18)

18.

A. Oncology is the department involved in the diagnosis and treatment of malignant (life-threatening) tumors. (p. 5)

19.

C. Phlebotomists must work with all other members of a health care team. (pp. 3–7)

20.

C. The department of gastroenterology deals with diseases and disorders related to the esophagus, stomach, and intestines. (p. 4)

21.

C. The nephrology department deals with disorders and diseases of the kidneys. (p. 5)

22.

C. Collecting a blood specimen is an example of the preanalytical phase of the clinical laboratory workflow pathway. It is the most important phase for phlebotomists. (p. 9)

23.

C. Typical laboratory departments have two components: clinical pathology and surgical or anatomic pathology. (p. 12)

24.

B. Ambulatory care refers to personal health care provided to an individual who is not bedridden and is mobile, therefore is an outpatient. (p. 3)

25.

B. Laboratory analysis is used for diagnosis, therapeutic assessment, and monitoring of patients' health status. Developing a community needs assessment can be very helpful to the overall community but does *not* fit the immediate health needs of an individual patient. (p. 2)

26.

D. The phlebotomist is involved in selecting and performing the appropriate quality control procedures such as monitoring the expiration dates on blood collection vacuum tubes. (p. 15)

27.

B. Phlebotomists play a vital role in the preanalytic phase of specimen collection, the part of the process that occurs before the actual testing and analysis is performed. The preanalytic process is the fundamental and crucial domain of every phlebotomist. (p. 9)

28.

A. The federal government (CMS) regulates all clinical laboratories through the CLIA '88. (p. 8)

The AABB has oversight only of clinical laboratories that have blood banking (transfusion medicine testing).

29.

A. Reporting final clinical laboratory test results is an example of the postanalytical phase of the clinical laboratory workflow pathway. (p. 9)

30.

B. Eating a balanced diet, getting enough rest and/or time for relaxation, and exercising outside of the workplace can contribute to lowered stress levels and a more positive outlook at work and in one's personal life. (pp. 21–22)

31.

C. For hygiene and safety reasons, shoulder-length (or longer) hair should be pulled back and secured. (p. 20)

32.

B. The otolaryngology department is involved in the diagnosis and treatment of disorders and diseases related to the ears, nose, and throat. (p. 6)

33.

C. Sandals or flip-flops are not recommended for phlebotomists due to safety concerns. Shoes should be comfortable, safe, clean, polished, and not noisy when walked in, and socks or hosiery should be worn. (p. 21)

34.

B. Six Sigma is a method or framework designed to improve process performance by reducing variation, improving quality, enhancing financial performance, and improving customer satisfaction. (p. 24)

35.

A. The neonatology department treats and supports the needs of newborn and prematurely born babies. (p. 5)

36.

B. The medical laboratory technician or clinical laboratory technician is typically an individual with a 2-year degree who performs designated laboratory testing, processing, and collecting of specimens. (p. 11)

37.

C. Waived tests are those tests that are easiest to perform and least risky to patients. They include urinalysis. The other answers were tests of moderate or high complexity. (p. 10)

38.

A. Health care workers can use four major categories to help frame the concept of "professionalism." These are: respect (personal appearance, confidentiality, courtesy, tolerance, effective communication), service (shifting focus from oneself to others, commitment to job duties), support (following organizational policies, clean work spaces, reporting damaged equipment, respectfully disagreeing), and growth (continuing education, learning more about people who work with you). (pp. 14–15)

39.

A. Productivity measures for phlebotomy services can include patient waiting time. It is a measure of efficiency. (p. 17)

40.

D. In a health care setting, anyone involved in the health care process inside the organization is a potential customer. This includes patients, family members, support groups, and all health care workers. Special interest groups may be considered external stake holders, for example, advocacy groups (AARP), insurance companies, agencies that provide funding. (p. 23)

41.

B. Routine checking of the temperature of a specimen refrigerator is an example of a quality control function. (p. 32)

42.

A. Geriatrics is the department that is specifically responsible for the diagnosis and treatment of othe elderly population. (p. 4)

43.

B. In the anatomic pathology area, autopsies are performed and surgical biopsy tissues are analyzed. (p. 7)

44.

C. Cytogenetics analysis and electrophoresis testing fall in the category of high-complexity tests, since they are complex to perform and may allow for reasonable risk of harm to the patient if the results are inaccurate. (p. 10)

45.

B. The PDCA (plan-do-check-act) cycle represents a strategy for quality improvement. It uses a cycle of *planning* the change, *doing* the improvement, *collecting* the data and analyzing the results, *checking* the results to see whether the change improved the situation, and *acting* on what was learned by rejecting , adjusting , or adopting the change as a standard part of the process. (p. 27)

46.

D. Cause-and-effect diagrams can be used in quality improvement methodologies and are designed to assist in identifying interactions among people, methods, equipment, and supplies. (pp. 27–28)

47.

A. Pareto charts can be used in quality improvement methodologies to show the frequency of problematic events. The Pareto principle suggests that 80% of the trouble comes from 20% of the problems. (pp. 27–28)

48.

A. Flowcharts can be used in quality improvement to break out components into a diagram for easier visualization and understanding of a process. (pp. 27–28)

49.

D. Quality improvement efforts for specimen collection frequently involve assessment of the phlebotomist's technique, frequency of hematomas, recollection rates, and/or multiple sticks on the same patient. Drug reactions, while important, are normally beyond the phlebotomist's scope of practice. (p. 26)

50.

A. Hematoma formation (frequency of occurrence and size) is an example of an outcome that can be assessed for quality improvement purposes. (p. 27)

CHAPTER

2 Communication, Computerization, and Documentation

chapter objectives

Upon completion of Chapter 2, the learner is responsible for the following:

1. Outline the basic communication loop.
2. Describe methods for effective verbal and nonverbal communication, active listening, and written communication.
3. List examples of positive and negative body language.
4. Describe methods to achieve cultural competence and sensitivity in the workplace.
5. Describe the basic components of the medical record.
6. Provide examples of maintaining confidentiality and privacy related to patient information.
7. Describe essential elements of laboratory test requisitions, specimen labels, and test results.
8. Identify potential clerical or technical errors that may occur during labeling or documentation of phlebotomy procedures.

9. Identify essential components and functions of computers in health care.
10. Describe ways that health care workers may use computer systems to accomplish job functions.

DIRECTIONS Each of the questions or incomplete statements below is followed by four suggested answers or completions. Select one answer that is best in each case.

1. Which of the following is the most effective form of communication?
   A. reprimands
   B. telephone conversations
   C. face-to-face conversations
   D. personal letters/memos

2. Some patients are intimidated when confronted with a health care worker they do not know. Which of the following strategies would encourage a shy patient to communicate with a new phlebotomist?
   A. Move the patient from a bed to a chair.
   B. Show empathy and use active listening skills.
   C. Avoid direct eye contact with the patient.
   D. Give them instructions on paper.

3. Why is it important for phlebotomists to enjoy communicating with patients?
   A. improves public opinion
   B. is good for business and the industry
   C. helps Medicaid eligibility
   D. improves the likelihood of effective quality care

4. When a phlebotomist builds a good "rapport" with a patient, what is he or she doing?
   A. moving the patient to a different position for comfort
   B. being courteous and showing interest to improve patient satisfaction
   C. providing feedback about the illness
   D. filing lab reports in the patient's medical record

5. If a phlebotomist walks into a patient's room that has a television on very loudly, what should be the first course of action prior to beginning the procedure?
   A. Turn off the television immediately.
   B. Ask the patient if it is okay to reduce the volume or turn the television off.
   C. Ignore the television and proceed with the procedure because it distracts the patient from the pain of the venipuncture.
   D. Ask a family member to turn the television off and step out of the room.

6. What should a phlebotomist do if a patient cannot speak English and the patient's 11-year-old child offers to translate for his parent during the initial patient encounter?

A. Never allow the child to translate for his parent.
B. Allow the child to translate during the critical parts of the procedure.
C. Get a translator or written instructions in the patient's native language.
D. Leave the room immediately without speaking to the patient so that the child will not misinterpret anything you say.

7. While setting up for a routine venipuncture, the patient asked the phlebotomist, "Will this hurt?" What is the most appropriate response?
   A. It doesn't hurt and only takes a few seconds anyway.
   B. It only hurts for one second.
   C. It will hurt a little, but it should be over quickly.
   D. It can be terribly uncomfortable for some patients, but for others it is a piece of cake.

8. Which of the following is the appropriate protocol for health care workers who are involved in specimen collection?
   A. Once the laboratory tests have been performed on a patient, the blood collector can discuss these with the patient and family.
   B. If the blood collector is a phlebotomy student, it is best not to inform the patient that he or she is a student, since it may make the patient nervous.
   C. If family members asked for information on their child's laboratory results, the blood collector should seek out those results to help the family.
   D. The blood collector should state that the patient's physician ordered blood to be collected for testing and that it would be best to discuss the laboratory tests with the physician.

9. A busy phlebotomist was in a hurry one morning when she quickly awakened her next patient and suddenly approached the patient for a routine venipuncture. The patient became visibly nervous, anxious, and refused to have her blood collected. Which of the following factors could explain the patient's reaction?
   A. The phlebotomist intruded into the patient's zone of comfort too quickly.
   B. The patient was overmedicated.
   C. This was a normal way to approach a patient and the patient's reaction was unjustified.
   D. The phlebotomist was too cheerful and happy.

10. Cultural sensitivity for phlebotomists involve learning about all except which of the following factors?
   A. values
   B. beliefs
   C. traditions and practices
   D. skin sensitivity to pain

11. Which of the following behaviors should the phlebotomist avoid in his or her patient care and blood collection activities?
   A. making a deep sigh when collecting the blood
   B. smiling when he or she is around the patient
   C. making eye contact with the patient
   D. maintaining relaxed hands, arms, and shoulders

12. Braille is defined as which of the following?
    A. high-pitched female voice
    B. writing system for sightless individuals
    C. legal documents from electronic medical records
    D. social networking system

13. When communicating with a patient who has a hearing impairment, the first step in preparation would be which of the following?
    A. Increase the pace of your speech.
    B. Increase the tone of your voice.
    C. Reduce external noise.
    D. Pull out a pen and paper.

14. Use of American Sign Language is important for which type of patients?
    A. pediatric
    B. geriatric
    C. deaf
    D. visually impaired

15. At the end of any specimen collection procedure, what is the final statement the phlebotomist should say to the patient?
    A. Have a great day.
    B. Thank you.
    C. I'm sure you're glad to see me leave.
    D. I'll be back tomorrow.

16. A phlebotomist has entered a hospital room and the patient is Eliza Smith. After the phlebotomist introduces himself or herself, what is the next question he or she should ask to confirm the name or identity of the patient?
    A. Could you please state your name and spell it for me?
    B. I need to confirm that you are Eliza Smith, right?
    C. Are you Eliza Smith?
    D. Can you please spell Eliza Smith?

17. Why is documentation of all clinical events important?
    A. to monitor quality and coordination of care
    B. so that only the patient's physician can access the information
    C. so that employees can get merit raises
    D. so that public information may be disclosed during a financial inquiry

18. A nurse stated to a phlebotomist that one of a patient's lab test results was a mistake. The nurse asked the phlebotomist to change the test result immediately. What should the phlebotomist do?
    A. Make the change immediately.
    B. Investigate the situation more thoroughly prior to taking action.
    C. Leave the test result as it is.
    D. Call Occupational Safety and Health Administration (OSHA).

19. When documenting errors in a paper-based medical record, which of the following statements is most appropriate?
    A. Errors should be erased or deleted.
    B. Errors should be reported to the patient's family.
    C. The phlebotomist should give his or her opinion about who made the mistake.
    D. Errors should not be erased, but noted and corrected.

20. If a phlebotomist wanted to look up details about specimen containers or tube requirements while on duty at his or her hospital, what would probably be the best source for the information?

A. infection control procedures
B. quality control (QC) procedures
C. safety manual
D. specimen collection manual

21. Like many laboratory departments, one hospital's policies did not allow release of information directly to patients. However, a patient made an emergency telephone call to the laboratory and asked a specific question about his or her own laboratory result. What was the most appropriate course of action for the phlebotomist?
    A. Using a professional tone of voice, provide the patient with the information requested.
    B. Using a professional tone of voice, follow the organization's directions about referring the patient to the appropriate person.
    C. Provide a detailed explanation of the reasons for the policy and report the situation to a supervisor.
    D. Place the caller on hold while seeking an exception to the rule.

22. A phlebotomist inadvertently overheard a conversation between a doctor and a patient about a medical condition that is unrelated to the specimen collection or laboratory testing process. What is the best course of action regarding the sharing of this information with other individuals in the hospital?
    A. The information can be shared since it was already shared with the doctor.
    B. The information is privileged and should not be shared.
    C. The information is medically related and can be shared with anyone in the hospital.
    D. The information is classified and should not be shared.

23. A phlebotomist was asked by a patient to fax test results to her home so she would not have to go back to the doctor. What is the most appropriate course of action for the phlebotomist?
    A. Follow the employer's policies regarding the use or transmission of lab results.
    B. Fax the test results only the first time.
    C. Refuse to fax the test results, but give the patient a verbal report.
    D. Fax the test results under the condition that the patient must return to her doctor.

24. Bar codes can be used in health care for patient identification purposes. Which of the following characterizes how bar codes are interpreted?
    A. The bars indicate pricing for laboratory procedures.
    B. Light and dark bands of varying widths represent alphanumeric symbols.
    C. They contain the name of the institution.
    D. They reveal the nature of each specimen.

25. The most efficient and accurate way of making labels for specimens is by:
    A. printing the physician's orders directly from a card file
    B. printing from a computerized system
    C. manually labeling the specimens as each one is drawn
    D. prelabeling all the tubes to be collected for the day

26. What is an "RFID"?
    A. blood test for rheumatoid factor
    B. urine test that must be transported on ice
    C. test code for a rapid screening test
    D. identification tag using silicon chips and a wireless receiver

27. What type of information *cannot* be converted into bar code symbols?
    A. supplies and equipment inventory
    B. laboratory test codes
    C. handwritten information
    D. date of birth (DOB) of patient

28. A phlebotomist noticed that new printed labels for laboratory specimens came with a smaller transfer label. What could this smaller label be used for?
    A. aliquot tubes, cuvettes, and microscope slides
    B. bandage for patient's finger
    C. medical record file
    D. chemical reagents

29. In designing a report/results form for laboratory results, which one of the listed elements is not required?
    A. patient and physician identification
    B. date and time of collection
    C. reference ranges
    D. patient and physician addresses

30. The use of an electronically generated blood drawing list or log sheet in a specimen collection area serves to:
    A. provide a record of specimens collected
    B. keep confidential information available
    C. keep track of employee productivity
    D. track QC of supplies/reagents

31. QC records do *not* include information about:
    A. employee health
    B. proper use and storage information
    C. expiration dates and stability information
    D. precision and accuracy of testing supplies/reagents

32. Bar codes in phlebotomy applications are not used for which one of the following?
    A. patient's arm preference
    B. specimen accession numbers, test codes
    C. product numbers, inventory expiration dates
    D. patient names, DOB, patient identification numbers

33. A "critical value" is a:
    A. radical test value
    B. term for all test results from the emergency room
    C. test result that may be life threatening
    D. static value

Questions 34 and 35 relate to the following case scenario:

Mary was a medical assistant in a family health clinic with a small laboratory. She had responsibilities in several areas, including answering the phone in the laboratory, drawing blood specimens, clerical duties, and assisting with laboratory testing. One morning when the clinic was particularly busy, she had collected blood specimens for numerous patients and tried to process them quickly so that they could be tested in a timely manner. When the phone rang, she was reluctant to answer it because she had almost finished processing a batch of specimens. It rang several times; then she hurried to pick it up and asked the individual to "hold please." She went back to finish processing the samples and forgot the person on hold. Later, she found out that the individual on hold was a doctor who was trying to request another test on a previously drawn sample.

34. What should Mary have said when she first answered the phone?
    A. Hold for just a moment, please.
    B. Please hold while I process a few specimens so that they will not be delayed.

C. Hello, this is the clinic laboratory. May I help you?
D. Hello, I am sorry that I cannot assist you now. Please call back.

35. Additional training would benefit Mary. Based on this incident, which of the following topics would be the highest priority for her continuing education?
A. customer service, communication, and time management
B. centrifugation and specimen transportation basics
C. team building
D. updated computer technology

36. Computers can be used in which of the phases of clinical laboratory workflow?
A. preanalytic/preexamination
B. analytic/examination
C. postanalytic/postexamination
D. preanalytic, analytic, postanalytic

37. What should a phlebotomist do if there are too many visitors in a patient's room when a blood specimen is to be collected STAT?
A. Report the situation to hospital administration.
B. Politely ask the visitors to step into the hall while the blood is collected.
C. Tell them it is an emergency and they need to leave immediately.
D. Inform the doctor in charge of the patient.

38. If a patient is having a private conversation with his or her physician when the phlebotomist shows up to collect a routine blood specimen, what should the phlebotomist do?
A. Politely ask the physician to leave.
B. Perform the procedure at a later time.
C. Perform the procedure while the physician is there.
D. Ask the patient what his or her preference is.

39. When sending/receiving email communication, which of the following should be avoided?
A. use of an autoreply message if you are going on vacation
B. use of symbols such as !!!
C. noting which messages are "priority"
D. trying to respond within 24 hours

40. Baby boomers are individuals who were born during which time period?
A. prior to the mid-1940s
B. 1940s–1964
C. 1965–1981
D. 1982–2000

41. Which generation of workers is used to a more hierarchical form of leadership?
A. veterans/traditionalists
B. boomers
C. generation X
D. millennials/generation Y

42. Generations of workers are used to different forms of feedback from their supervisors and peers. Which group would most likely want instant feedback?
A. veterans/traditionalists
B. boomers
C. generation X
D. millennials/generation Y

43. Which group of workers would most likely be happy with little or no feedback, for example, "no news is good news"?
    A. veterans/traditionalists
    B. boomers
    C. generation X
    D. millennials/generation Y

44. When communicating with patients, changing one's speech to a faster pace and higher pitch can communicate a sense of:
    A. urgency and emergency
    B. relaxation and control
    C. confidence and calm
    D. sadness and depression

45. A moderate pace and volume in one's voice can communicate a sense of:
    A. urgency and emergency
    B. relaxation and control
    C. confidence and calm
    D. sadness and depression

46. A legally blind patient is entitled to use which of the following in any health care facility?
    A. satellite radio
    B. guide dog
    C. internet connection
    D. iPhone

47. Considering nonverbal communication, which of the following features is the most expressive part of the human face?
    A. forehead
    B. mouth
    C. eyes
    D. laugh lines

48. The term "critical value" refers to which of the following?
    A. a random laboratory result
    B. HIPAA regulation
    C. a life threatening test result
    D. a static test result

49. What type of laboratory test result should be reported to a patient's physician as soon as possible?
    A. all routine test results
    B. a critical value
    C. a CLIA waived test result
    D. a QC value that is not in range

50. Clinical or medical records, whether they are electronic or paper-based documents, provide legal protection because:
    A. they are open to the public for review
    B. they allow for research results on new drug therapies
    C. they provide proof that an action was performed and documented
    D. all employees can eliminate any errors found in the record

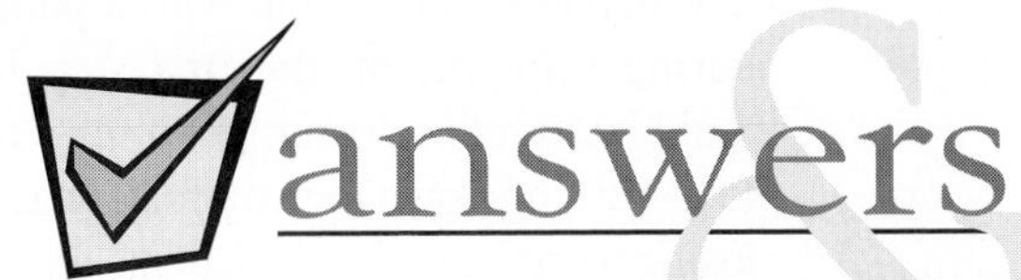

answers & rationales

1.

C. The most effective method of communication is through face-to-face conversations. (p. 41)

2.

B. Phlebotomists can encourage patients to communicate with them by showing empathy for them, building trust, establishing rapport, active listening, and providing feedback during the conversation. (p. 41)

3.

D. Communication is a vital part of a phlebotomist's job role and does help improve public opinion; however, there are other reasons that are more important for having positive communication skills. It is important for phlebotomists to take pleasure in communicating with patients because it improves the likelihood that the collection process will be successful and that the care given will be effective and of high quality. (p. 41)

4.

B. Building "rapport" involves developing a comfortable bond between the patient and the phlebotomist and involves common courtesy, showing interest in the patient, and building trust so as to improve communication and patient satisfaction. (p. 41)

5.

B. If the television is too loud, it can be a harmful distraction by preventing the patient from hearing the instructions about the procedure. In most cases, simply lowering the volume will alleviate the negative distraction (noise), yet allow the patient to have something to look at while enduring the procedure. As a courteous gesture, the patient should be asked if he or she mind reducing the volume, using the mute function, or turning the television off completely prior to performing the procedure. (p. 43)

6.

C. In some states, children are not permitted to serve as translators for their parents when health care issues are discussed. Phlebotomists should be knowledgeable of the applicable laws and their organization's policies and practices regarding translations. In many larger organizations, there are personnel available to assist with translations; additionally, online translation services and/or written instructions in languages other than English can be made available. (pp. 43–46)

7.

C. This is a truthful and accurate answer and demonstrates to the patient that it is only a temporary discomfort. (p. 58)

8.

D. The blood collector should state that the patient's physician ordered blood to be collected for testing and that it would be best to discuss the laboratory test with the physician. It is beyond the phlebotomist's scope of practice to interpret laboratory results. (p. 58)

9.

A. When a stranger gets too close, it can cause the patient to feel nervous, fearful, or anxious. The phlebotomist should have slowed down, gently awakened the patient, then calmly explained the purpose for interrupting her sleep. The phlebotomist intruded into the patient's zone of comfort and did so too quickly. (p. 53)

10.

D. Culture encompasses values, beliefs, traditions, and practices of a group of individuals. It is important that health care workers demonstrate cultural sensitivity toward patients from cultures different from their own. Skin sensitivity is not part of cultural sensitivity. (pp. 53–54)

11.

A. The phlebotomist should avoid making deep sighs around patients, since this can convey a feeling of being bored. (p. 52)

12.

B. Braille is defined as a writing system for sightless individuals. It consists of patterns of raised dots that are read by touch. (p. 48)

13.

C. When communicating with a patient who has a hearing impairment, the first step in preparation would be to reduce external noise as much as possible by turning down the volume of a radio/television, closing a door, etc. Some patients are not completely deaf and a quick assessment by the phlebotomist can help with further communication. (p. 46)

14.

C. American Sign Language may be considered as the first language for deaf patients while English may be the second language. Some deaf patients also have mild vision impairments but can still read sign language. If a deaf patient requests a sign-language interpreter, the health care provider must comply with this request. (p. 51)

15.

B. Under normal circumstances, after the specimen collection procedure, a phlebotomist should say a simple "thank you" for the patient's cooperation. (p. 58)

16.

A. After greeting a hospital patient and introducing herself, the phlebotomist should ask "Could you please state your name and spell it for me? Sometimes the exact wording may vary; however, the phlebotomist should *not* state the patient's name, for example, "Are you Eliza Smith?" because it is less reliable in confirming identification.

17.

A. Documentation of all clinical events is important for monitoring the quality of care given to the patient, for coordination of care among members of the health care team, for complying with accrediting and licensing standards, for providing legal protection, and in some cases for research purposes. (p. 69)

18.

B. Records should never be changed or altered to cover up a mistake. Errors should be noted according to the institution's policies. Generally speaking, the phlebotomist should investigate the situation and report it to a supervisor to identify the causes for the mistake (if it really is one) and take all corrective actions. (p. 71)

19.

D. When documenting errors in a paper-based medical record, errors should never be erased or deleted. The error should be noted according to the organization's protocol along with the corrected information. Typically, this involves marking a single line through the incorrect information (so that it can still be read) and writing the word "Error" with authorized initials. (p. 71)

20.

D. Specimen collection manuals, either electronic or paper versions, contain information about patient preparation, specimen containers, specimen tube requirements, timing requirements, preservative and anticoagulants, special handling or transportation needs, and clinical information needed for specific tests. (p. 72)

21.

B. Health care organizations have strict policies and procedures about releasing patient information. The phlebotomist should never release information unless authorized to do so. In this case, the phlebotomist was justified in politely and professionally referring the patient to an appropriate person who is authorized to counsel the patient and/or provide the requested information. (p. 73)

22.

B. Patient information should not be shared with individuals who are not directly involved in the care of a patient without prior consent of the patient. In this case, the communication that was overheard is considered privileged and private. (p. 73)

23.

A. Health Insurance Portability and Accountability Act (HIPAA) laws apply to fax transmissions even though the use of electronic transmissions is a timely way of communicating. However, patients' permissions are needed to disclose information and each facility should have policies related to the use of electronic transmissions. (p. 63)

24.

B. When describing bar code usage for patient identification purposes, they are interpreted by using light and dark bands of varying widths that represent alphanumeric symbols (i.e., a name and number). (pp. 65–66)

25.

A. The most accurate method to generate specimen labels is by using electronic/computer systems because manual labeling systems are time consuming and prone to transcription errors. Computerization of the collection process can significantly decrease errors because data are continually being checked against the computer files, and authorized individuals can add to and receive designated information. (p. 67)

26.

D. RFID, radio frequency identification, is another form of identification tag that is used for identifying and tracking records, specimens, patients, equipment, and supplies. It uses a silicon chip that transmits data to a wireless receiver. (p. 65)

27.

C. Handwritten information cannot be directly barcoded. (p. 65)

28.

A. Small printed transfer labels can be used for aliquot tubes, cuvettes, and microscope slides. (pp. 64, 67)

29.

D. CAP recommends that in designing a laboratory report form, the following issues should be considered: identification of patient and physician, patient location, date and time of specimen collection, source and description of specimen, precautions, packaging requirements for the specimen, understandability of the report, ability to be located in the patient's clinical record, reference ranges, and abnormal values. Patient and physician addresses are *not* required. (p. 202)

30.

A. A blood drawing list, or log sheet, can serve to provide a record of specimens that have been collected throughout the day. For hospital use, a copy could be located on a nursing unit as well as in the laboratory. (p. 193)

31.

A. QC information usually contains facts about the following: hazards associated with the use of a reagent or supplies, proper use and storage information, expiration dates and stability information, and indications for measuring the precision and accuracy of the analytical process to be involved. Employee health information is *not* normally included in QC data. (p. 73)

32.

A. Bar codes have not been used to determine the patient's arm preferences. However, they have many applications in specimen identification, processing, and testing, including patient names, DOB, identification numbers, test codes, accession numbers, billing codes, product numbers, and inventory records. (p. 65)

33.

C. A "critical value" is a test result that may be life threatening and must be reported immediately to the patient's physician. (pp. 68–69)

34.

C. Mary should have stopped her work temporarily to answer the phone or asked for assistance. If she had no assistance, she should have greeted the caller in a polite and professional manner, stated the department name, and asked how she could help. She should have restated the request or asked for clarification and documented it. (p. 49)

35.

A. Customer service and time management are critical aspects of any job in health care. And, the telephone is one of the most frequently used methods of live communication in a busy clinic. It is vitally important that health care workers be aware of the procedures for operating it and the etiquette for professional dialogue. Mary's training should include effective customer service manners, transferring calls, placing someone on hold, using an intercom system, using voice mail, organizing conference calls, using speakerphones, documenting complete messages, and appropriate greetings. In this case, Mary seems to have a working knowledge of the processing techniques that most likely include centrifugation. Therefore, the focus of her training should be those mentioned earlier. (p. 49)

36.

D. Computers are used in all phases of laboratory testing. (p. 61)

37.

B. When there are too many visitors in the patient's room, the phlebotomist can politely ask them to step into the hallway for a short time while the procedure is performed. (p. 58)

38.

B. If a patient is having a private conversation with his or her physician when the phlebotomist shows up to collect a routine blood specimen, the phlebotomist should respect that private conversation and return at a later time to collect the specimen. (p. 49)

39.

B. When using email communications, the use of excessive symbols such as !!! and ??? should be avoided because they are confusing, the meaning is unclear, and they may be read as offensive. (p. 50)

40.

B. Baby boomers are individuals born between the mid-1940s and 1964. (pp. 45–46)

41.

A. Veterans/traditionalists/matures are used to a more hierarchical form of leadership. (pp. 45–46)

42.

D. Millennials/Internet/generation Y workers would most likely want instant feedback on their work. (pp. 44–45)

43.

A. Veterans/traditionalists/mature workers would most likely want little or no feedback. (pp. 44–45)

44.

A. High pitched, rapid voices communicate a sense of urgency. (p. 47)

45.

C. A moderate pace and volume in one's voice can communicate a sense of calm, confidence, and professionalism. (p. 47)

46.

B. A legally blind patient is entitled to use a long white cane or guide dog to walk independently. (p. 50)

47.

C. The eyes are the most expressive part of the human face. Eye contact can convey a sense of trust and honesty among workers and patients. (p. 51)

48.

D. A critical value is a laboratory test result that may be potentially life-threatening and must be reported to the patient's physician in a timely manner. (pp. 68–69)

49.

B. A critical value is a laboratory test result that may be potentially life-threatening and must be reported to the patient's physician in a timely manner. (pp. 68–69)

50.

C. Clinical or medical records provide proof that an action was performed and documented. They serve as supporting evidence in legal cases. If a health care worker does not record what occurred, or is incomplete in the documentation of a procedure, then it can be assumed that the procedure was not performed or done incorrectly. (p. 70)

CHAPTER

3 Professional Ethics, Legal, and Regulatory Issues

chapter objectives

Upon completion of Chapter 3, the learner is responsible for the following:

1. Define basic ethical and legal terms and explain how they differ.
2. Describe types of consent used in health care settings, including *informed consent* and *implied consent.*
3. Describe how to avoid litigation as it relates to blood collection.
4. Define *standard of care* from a legal and a health care provider's perspective.
5. Identify key elements of the *Health Insurance Portability and Accountability Act* (HIPAA).
6. List key factors common to health professional liability insurance policies.
7. List common issues in lawsuits against health care providers and prevention tips to avoid lawsuits in phlebotomy.

DIRECTIONS Each of the questions or incomplete statements below is followed by four suggested answers or completions. Select one answer that is best in each case.

1. Moral issues or problems that have occurred because of the latest medical research and/or technology are described as:
   a. executive law
   b. patient's Bill of Rights
   c. bioethics
   d. judicial law

2. In past research studies, the unethical treatment of humans led to:
   A. The Joint Commission
   B. HIPAA
   C. The National Research Act
   D. JCAHO

3. When "a patient should be allowed to die" is a topic closely related to:
   A. the executive branch of the government
   B. moral issues of bioethics
   C. negligence
   D. criminal law

4. A large number of negligence health care lawsuit cases arise out of the violation of:
   A. CMS requirements
   B. statutes made at the state level
   C. statutes made at the federal level
   D. privacy of patient confidentiality

5. An agency that has recognized patient's rights through the *Patient Care Partnership* is:
   A. CLIA '88
   B. American Hospital Association (AHA)
   C. Joint Commission on Accreditation of Healthcare Organizations (JCAHO)
   D. CMS

6. A phlebotomist performing which of the following procedures is considered a CLIA '88-waived procedure?
   A. venipuncture for a donor blood transfusion
   B. dipstick urinalysis
   C. fingerstick blood collection for a reticulocyte count
   D. venipuncture for a WBC

7. Bioethics refers to:
   A. protecting the safety of societal integrity
   B. "life-and-death" issues
   C. moral standards of behavior
   D. societal rules and regulations

8. Cross-examination is:
   A. the same as a deposition
   B. used immediately when a malpractice lawsuit is filed
   C. used during the trial to obtain information regarding the possibility of malpractice of a health care worker or in other types of trials as well
   D. used before the trial to obtain medical records and laboratory test results to determine negligence of a health care worker

9. If the phlebotomist unintentionally hit the patient's median nerve in the venipuncture procedure, he or she
   A. is a felon
   B. has committed a crime
   C. can be accused of professional negligence
   D. will be handed a misdemeanor charge

10. A child who refused to have his blood collected was locked in a room by a health care worker and was forced to have his blood collected. This is an example of:
    A. informed consent
    B. invasion of privacy
    C. assault and battery
    D. a misdemeanor

11. The best definition for ethics is:
    A. societal rules or regulations
    B. moral standards of behavior
    C. societal protection of the public
    D. conflict resolution through regulations

12. All of the following are ways to avoid malpractice litigation *except:*
    A. regularly participating in continuing education programs
    B. reporting incidents within 48 hours
    C. properly handling all confidential communications without violation
    D. obtaining consent for collection of specimens

13. If a phlebotomist has a lawsuit filed against him or her, he or she is the
    A. plaintiff
    B. defendant
    C. respondeat superior
    D. prosecutor

14. If a phlebotomist makes a statement that is false regarding a patient, his or her action is:
    A. respondeat superior
    B. breach of duty
    C. malice
    D. battery

15. Before a patient's laboratory test results can legally be released, the patient must:
    A. provide verbal permission
    B. tell his or her physician or nurse practitioner that it is okay
    C. provide written consent
    D. provide his or her lawyer's consent

16. Which legal concept refers to the voluntary permission by a patient to allow touching, examination, and/or treatment by health care providers?
    A. implied consent
    B. standard of care
    C. informed consent
    D. assault and battery

17. An IRB requires:
    A. implied consent of the research participant
    B. a blood collector in a research project to attend a course on the protection of research participants
    C. a statute of limitations
    D. interpreters be present for the implied consent

18. In HIV-related issues for phlebotomists, the
    A. employee is legally responsible for monitoring HIV post-exposure follow-up
    B. incident report at the health care facility is not usually involved in legal issues
    C. employer is legally responsible for monitoring HIV post-exposure follow-up
    D. phlebotomist contracting AIDS during work will not be covered for health care if he or she discontinues work

19. The CLIA '88 was passed to:
    A. provide malpractice insurance coverage for laboratory personnel, including phlebotomists
    B. ensure the quality and accuracy of nursing care in health care facilities
    C. ensure the quality and accuracy of laboratory testing
    D. ensure that HIV testing occurred on all laboratory personnel

20. Malpractice phlebotomy cases lead to decisions primarily made in what branch of government?
    A. legislative branch of the state government
    B. executive branch
    C. judicial branch
    D. legislative branch of the federal government

21. For a phlebotomist to collect blood for a research study in a health care institution, he or she must obtain consent from the research participant due to:
    A. standard of care
    B. IRB requirements
    C. the AHA requirements
    D. CLIA '88 requirements

22. A patient claimed in court that the phlebotomist did not perform proper blood collection procedure that led to an alleged injury. The patient must show that the phlebotomist failed to meet:
    A. the criminal laws in the state
    B. the prevailing standard of care
    C. the administrative laws of the state
    D. HIPAA requirements

23. In alleged negligence cases when "the plaintiff must be able to show what actually happened and that the defendant acted unreasonably," what factor does this indicate?
    A. breach of duty
    B. proximate causation
    C. damages
    D. foreseeability

24. Violation of patient confidentiality:
    A. can be considered professional negligence
    B. is considered only in CLIA '88's moderately complex procedures
    C. is considered respondeat superior
    D. can be considered assault and battery

25. When should incident reports involving accidental HIV exposures be reported?
    A. at the end of the work shift
    B. immediately
    C. after 24 hours
    D. after seeing the employee health physician

26. Which federal agency or act states that a laboratory with moderately complex or highly complex testing must have written policies and procedures for specimen collection and labeling?
    A. Food and Drug Administration (FDA)
    B. Health Care Financing Administration (HCFA)
    C. Environmental Protection Agency (EPA)
    D. CLIA '88

27. The legal term for improper or unskillful care of a patient by a member of the health care team or any professional misconduct, unreasonable lack of skill, or infidelity in professional or judiciary duties is:
    A. malpractice
    B. misdemeanor
    C. litigation
    D. liability

28. Which of the following legal branches writes laws called statutes?
    A. legislative branch
    B. judicial branch
    C. U.S. Supreme Court
    D. executive branch

29. The judicial branch of the government:
    A. establishes written statutes to control immoral acts
    B. establishes case law
    C. provides administrative laws based on legal cases
    D. uses legal cases to establish written statutes

30. Which of the following legal terms refers to the concept that supervisors and directors may be held liable for the negligent actions of their employees?
    A. malice
    B. respondeat superior
    C. *res ipsa loquitur*
    D. misdemeanor

31. The phrase "if you do not let me collect your blood, your infection will probably become severe" spoken by a phlebotomist to a patient can:
    A. lead to false imprisonment
    B. lead to an assault and battery charge
    C. create a situation in which the phlebotomist becomes a plaintiff against the patient
    D. create a lawsuit under the HIPAA regulations

32. What is cross-examination in malpractice lawsuits?
    A. information obtained during the trial to obtain information regarding the possibility of malpractice of a health care worker.
    B. the testimony of an expert witness in a deposition regarding the possibility of malpractice of a health care worker
    C. information obtained before the trial to obtain information regarding the possibility of malpractice of a health care worker
    D. the same as a deposition

33. Mrs. Harriott, a phlebotomist who collects blood in Valley View Hospital from 6:00 A.M. to 12:00 P.M. during the week must annually review and sign a confidentiality and nondisclosure agreement that describes the sensitivity of patient information due to which of the following acts?
    A. FDA
    B. HIPAA
    C. PHI
    D. OSHA

34. If a phlebotomist gives his or her friend the results of a patient's HIV test results, what can be claimed by the patient against the phlebotomist?
    A. assault
    B. battery
    C. negligence
    D. misdemeanor

35. Examination of witnesses before and/or during a trial is referred to as:
    A. discovery
    B. statute of limitation
    C. respondent superior
    D. implied consent

36. Which of the following refers to the testimony of a witness that has been recorded in a written legal format?
    A. medical records
    B. deposition
    C. statute of limitations
    D. documentation of communication between the physician and the health care team

37. The largest area of litigation regarding health care workers (including phlebotomists) is the:
    A. statute of limitations
    B. implied consent principle
    C. negligence
    D. FDA requirements

38. Which of the following is the best example of setting the standard of care for blood collection?
    A. Texas Association of Clinical Laboratory Sciences
    B. Southwest Regional Phlebotomists' Association
    C. California Clinical Laboratory Association
    D. AHA

39. Professional negligence in blood collection is the same as:
    A. malice
    B. malpractice
    C. informed consent
    D. implied consent

40. When a health care provider gives aid at an accident, he or she is usually protected through:
    A. informed consent
    B. implied consent
    C. CLIA '88
    D. rightful action consent

41. Failure to act or perform duties according to the standards of the profession is:
    A. battery
    B. negligence
    C. criminal action
    D. slander

42. Which of the following agencies requires an inspection for quality laboratory testing?
    A. FDA
    B. EPA
    C. OSHA
    D. CLIA '88

43. A national organization that develops guidelines and safety measures and sets national standards that affect laboratory professionals is the:
    A. New York Licensure Department for Medical Laboratory Sciences
    B. JCAHO
    C. AHA
    D. Texas Department of Health and Human Services

44. The term PHI was actually created by which of the following?
    A. CDC
    B. HIPAA

C. CLIA ’88
D. AHA

45. In legal cases, “what a reasonably prudent person would do under similar circumstances” refers to:
A. discovery
B. standard of care
C. informed consent
D. implied consent

46. During a patient’s appointment with his physician, he fills out the necessary legal papers and meets with his physician. After his physical exam, the physician orders laboratory tests for diagnosis and the patient comes to the laboratory with a rolled-up sleeve. The patient is giving:
A. implied consent
B. informed consent
C. rightful action consent
D. preventive consent

47. Misidentifying the patient, which can lead to confusion of patients’ samples and possible wrong diagnosis and death, is considered:
A. assault
B. negligence
C. battery
D. a HIPAA violation

48. The standard of care currently used in phlebotomy malpractice legal cases involving health care providers is based on the conduct of the average health care provider in which area?
A. city
B. state
C. national community
D. regional community

49. Which of the following organizations is influential in setting the “standard of care” for phlebotomy practice?
A. EPA
B. IRB
C. The Joint Commission
D. HIPAA

50. The federal law enacted that regulates the quality and accuracy of laboratory testing (including phlebotomy procedures) by creating a uniform set of provisions governing all clinical laboratories is referred to as:
A. HCFA
B. FDA
C. CLIA ’88
D. The Joint Commission

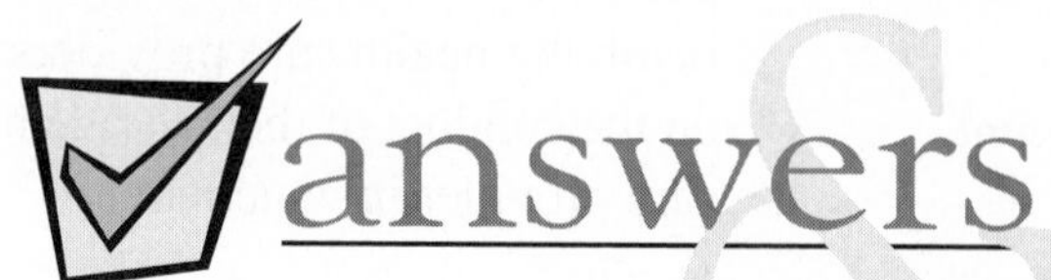

answers & rationales

1.

C. Bioethics ("bio" means "life") refers to the moral issues or problems that have resulted because of modern medicine, clinical research, and/or technology. (p. 82)

2.

C. As a result of unethical treatment of humans in the past for research purposes, the United States passed a law in 1974, the National Research Act. (p. 89)

3.

B. Bioethics refers to "life-and-death" issues. (p. 82)

4.

D. Negligence cases can arise out of violation of the right to privacy or violation of patient confidentiality. (p. 87)

5.

B. The AHA has recognized rights for patients in health care organizations through the *Patient Care Partnership*. (p. 83)

6.

B. The dipstick urinalysis is a CLIA '88-waived laboratory procedure. (p. 96)

7.

B. Bioethics is the study of moral issues or problems that refer to "life-and-death" issues such as abortion, when a patient should be allowed to die, etc. (p. 82)

8.

C. Cross-examination occurs during the trial that relates to the accusation of the malpractice that occurred by the health care worker. It is *not* used immediately when a lawsuit is filed. (p. 91)

9.

C. If the phlebotomist unintentionally hit the patient's median nerve during a venipuncture procedure, he or she can be accused of professional negligence. (p. 94)

10.

C. Assault is the unjustifiable attempt to touch another person or threaten to do so in such circumstances as to cause the other to believe it will be carried out. Battery is the intentional touching of another person without consent and the unlawful beating of another or carrying out of the threatened physical harm (i.e., blood collection without consent). (p. 85)

11.

B. Ethics refers to the moral standards of behavior or conduct that govern an individual's actions. (p. 82)

12.

B. To avoid malpractice litigation, it is extremely important to:

- obtain consent for collection of specimens
- regularly participate in continuing education programs
- report incidents immediately and document them
- properly handle all confidential communications without violation. (p. 93)

13.

B. If a phlebotomist has a lawsuit filed against him or her, he or she is the defendant. (p. 84)

14.

C. If a phlebotomist makes a statement that is false regarding a patient, this action is malice. (p. 85)

15.

C. Before a patient's laboratory test results can legally be released, the patient must provide written consent. (pp. 88–89)

16.

C. Informed consent refers to the voluntary permission by a patient to allow touching, examination, and/or treatment by health care providers. (pp. 88–89)

17.

B. An IRB requires the blood collector in a research project to attend a course on the protection of research participants. (pp. 89–90)

18.

C. In HIV-related issues for phlebotomists, the employer is legally responsible for monitoring HIV post-exposure follow-up. (pp. 87–88)

19.

C. The CLIA '88 was passed to ensure the quality and accuracy of laboratory testing. (p. 96)

20.

C. Malpractice phlebotomy cases lead to decisions primarily made in the judicial branch of government. (p. 83)

21.

B. The IRBs at institutions (e.g., hospitals, universities) require that any research project utilizing human subjects requires the informed consent of those subjects prior to their participation. (pp. 89–90)

22.

B. If a patient has suffered injury due to blood collection, the patient must show that the health care worker who collected the blood failed to meet the prevailing standard of care. (p. 88)

23.

A. Five factors must be considered in alleged negligence cases and the second one, breach of duty, indicates that "the plaintiff must be able to show what actually happened and that the defendant acted unreasonably." (p. 86)

24.

A. Violation of patient confidentiality can be considered professional negligence. (p. 87)

25.

B. An incident report involving accidental HIV exposure should be reported immediately. Actually, any blood collection incident needs to be reported immediately. (p. 93)

26.

D. The CLIA '88 is the act over clinical laboratory testing that has written policies and procedures for specimen collection and labeling. (p. 96)

27.

A. Malpractice is defined as improper or unskillful care of a patient by a member of the health care team or any professional misconduct or unreasonable lack of skill. (p. 86)

28.

A. The legislative branch of government develops written laws, called statutes, that are made at the federal, state, and county levels. (p. 83)

29.

B. The function of the judicial branch of the local, state, and federal government is to resolve disputes in accordance with the law, and thus, establishes case laws. (p. 83)

30.

B. Respondeat superior refers to the concept that supervisors and directors may be held liable for the negligent actions of their employees. (p. 85)

31.

B. The phrase "if you do not let me collect your blood, your infection will probably become severe" spoken by a phlebotomist to a patient can lead to an assault and battery charge. (p. 84)

32.

A. Cross-examination is information obtained during the trial regarding the possibility of malpractice of a health care worker. (p. 91)

33.

B. HIPAA created legal requirements for the protection, security, and appropriate sharing of a patient's personal health information. (p. 86)

34.

C. Negligence can be claimed if the patient's HIV test results are released to anyone other than the attending physician or other authorized individual. (pp. 85–86)

35.

A. In legal terms, discovery is the right to examine the witness before and/or during the trial. (p. 91)

36.

B. The deposition is the testimony of a witness that has been recorded in a written legal format. (p. 91)

37.

C. The largest area of litigation regarding health care workers (including phlebotomists) is negligence in using improper or unskillful technique or care of a patient. (p. 94)

38.

D. All health care workers must conform to a specific standard of care to protect patients. In legal cases, the standard of care represents the conduct of the average health care worker in the community. The community has been expanded to the national community and is based on rules and regulations established by national professional organizations. (p. 88)

39.

B. Professional negligence is the improper or unskillful care of a patient by a member of the health care team and is usually referred to as malpractice. (p. 86)

40.

B. Implied consent exists when immediate action is required to save a patient's life. (p. 90)

41.

B. Failure to act or perform duties according to the standards of the profession is negligence. (p. 86)

42.

D. In October 1988, the U.S. Congress passed the CLIA'88. The law is referred to as CLIA '88 and became effective in 1992 as a means to ensure the quality and accuracy of laboratory testing (including blood collection) and requires inspection for quality laboratory testing. (p. 96)

43.

C. All health care workers must conform to a specific standard of care to protect patients. In legal cases, the standard of care represents the conduct of the average health care worker in the community. The community has been expanded to the national community and is based on rules and regulations established by national professional organizations such as the AHA that has developed guidelines (i.e., Patient Care Partnership). (pp. 83, 88)

44.

B. HIPAA created legal requirements for the protection, security, and appropriate sharing of a patient's personal health information referred to as "PHI." (p. 86)

45.

B. In legal cases, the standard of care is determined by what a reasonably prudent person would do under similar circumstances. (p. 88)

46.

B. Informed consent is voluntary permission by a patient to allow touching, examination, and/or treatment by health care providers. It allows patients to determine what will be performed on or to their bodies. By voluntarily rolling up his sleeve, the patient was allowing the health care provider to collect his blood. (pp. 88–89)

47.

B. Misidentifying the patient, which can lead to confusion of patients' samples and possible wrong diagnosis and death, is considered negligence. (p. 86)

48.

C. The standard of care currently used in phlebotomy malpractice legal cases and other health care malpractice legal cases is based on the national community as a result of national standards and requirements. (p. 88)

49.

C. The Joint Commission oversees the accreditation of health care organizations nationally and, thus, sets a national "standard of care" for phlebotomy practice. (p. 88)

50.

C. In October 1988, the U.S. Congress passed the CLIA '88. The law is referred to as CLIA '88 and became effective in 1992 as a means to ensure the quality and accuracy of laboratory testing (including blood collection). (p. 96)

CHAPTER

4 Infection Control

chapter objectives

Upon completion of Chapter 4, the learner is responsible for the following:

1. Explain the infection control policies and procedures that must be followed in specimen collection and transportation.
2. Define the terms *health–care–associated, health–care–acquired,* and *nosocomial infections*.
3. Identify the basic programs for infection control and isolation procedures.
4. Explain the proper techniques for handwashing, gowning, gloving, masking, double bagging, and entering and exiting the various isolation areas.
5. Identify steps to avoid transmission of blood-borne pathogens.
6. Identify ways to reduce risks for infections and accidental needlesticks.
7. Describe measures that can break each link in the chain of infection.
8. Identify the steps to be taken in the case of blood-borne pathogen exposure.

DIRECTIONS Each of the questions or incomplete statements below is followed by four suggested answers or completions. Select one answer that is best in each case.

1. Which of the following is a commonly identified pathogenic microorganism that causes health-care-acquired skin infections?
   A. *Haemophilus vaginalis*
   B. *Candida albicans*
   C. *Haemophilus influenzae*
   D. *Moraxella lacunata*

2. The clinical laboratory contributes to all of the following *except:*
   A. evaluating the effectiveness of sterilization or decontamination procedures
   B. decontaminating the surgery rooms with disinfectants to kill amebic organisms
   C. reporting on infectious agents and drug-resistant microorganisms
   D. maintaining laboratory records for surveillance purposes

3. Transmission-based precautions to reduce the spread of meningitis are referred to as:
   A. contact precautions
   B. complete isolation precautions
   C. airborne precautions
   D. droplet precautions

4. After completion of blood collection in an isolation room, which of the following steps should occur last?
   A. Remove the gloves.
   B. Remove the mask.
   C. Wash hands.
   D. Remove the gown.

5. An outbreak of particular health-care-acquired infections in a health care facility is detected through:
   A. the clinical chemistry department
   B. infection control surveillance
   C. personnel records
   D. individuals transmitting fomites

6. Health-care-acquired infections occur when what is complete?
   A. infection control surveillance
   B. an employee health monitoring program
   C. chain of infection
   D. a nosocomial infection

7. Health-care-acquired infections are also referred to as:
   A. nonpathogenic
   B. bloodborne pathogens
   C. nosocomial infections
   D. aseptic

8. A commonly identified causative agent of health-care-acquired infections in the nursery unit is:
   A. *Escherichia coli*
   B. *Shigella*
   C. *Vibrio cholerae*
   D. *Haemophilus vaginalis*

9. In the process of preparing to enter a patient's room in isolation, which of the following would occur first?
   A. donning gloves and positioning them
   B. donning mask
   C. discarding mask
   D. untying gown at the neck

10. Antiseptics for skin include:
   A. hypochlorite solution
   B. formaldehyde
   C. ethylene oxide
   D. iodine

11. Which of the following organizations requires the development and implementation of an infection control program in a health care facility?
   A. ASCP
   B. CLT
   C. CLIA '88
   D. The Joint Commission

12. What, as part of the U.S. Public Health Service, oversees the investigation of various diseases?
   A. Clinical Laboratory Standards Institute (CLSI)
   B. FDA
   C. Centers for Disease Control and Prevention (CDC)
   D. The Joint Commission

13. A nosocomial infection occurs when:
   A. the chain of infection is complete
   B. a source is detected
   C. a means of transmission is maintained by disinfectants
   D. a susceptible host remains stable

14. The following hand-hygiene antiseptic agent is most effective for *Mycobacterium tuberculosis:*
   A. iodophors
   B. isopropyl alcohol
   C. phenol
   D. quaternary ammonium

15. Which of the following is a commonly occurring pathogenic agent that causes health-care-acquired (nosocomial) infections of the gastrointestinal tract?
   A. *Haemophilus vaginalis*
   B. *Vibrio cholerae*
   C. *Neisseria gonorrhoeae*
   D. *Bordetella pertussis*

16. The label shown in Figure 4.1 will most likely be posted in the entrance to the:
   A. nuclear medicine department
   B. radiation therapy department
   C. TB culture area
   D. clinical chemistry area

FIGURE 4.1

17. Which of the following chemical compounds is an antiseptic for skin?
    A. hexylresorcinol
    B. ethylene oxide
    C. 1% phenol
    D. chlorophenol

18. Which of the following interrupts the link between the susceptible host and the source in the chain of infection?
    A. gene splicing
    B. radiation therapy
    C. chemotherapy
    D. good nutrition

19. Protective isolation is commonly used for patients who have:
    A. cholera
    B. hepatitis B
    C. immunodeficiency disorders
    D. whooping cough

20. Of the 35 million patients admitted to hospitals annually in the United States, about how many acquire a nosocomial infection?
    A. 0.25–0.5 million
    B. 0.5–1.0 million
    C. 1.75–3 million
    D. 5–6.5 million

21. Which of the following illnesses is usually transmitted from one person to another by coughing or sneezing?
    A. scabies
    B. weeping dermatitis
    C. diphtheria
    D. impetigo caused by *Staphylococcus*

22. A phlebotomist had to avoid contact with patients for 24 hours after being started on an appropriate antibiotic and appearing symptom-free. What type of infection could he or she have acquired for such work limitations to apply?
    A. measles
    B. strep throat (group A)
    C. chicken pox
    D. rubella

23. The warning label in Figure 4.2 was originally established as a requirement by:
    A. CLIA '88
    B. OSHA
    C. ASCP
    D. FDA

FIGURE 4.2

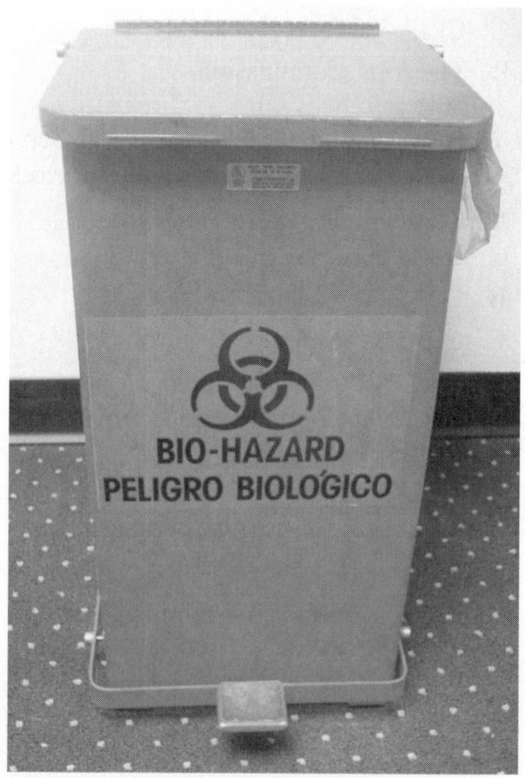

24. Under the CDC isolation guidelines, three sets of precautions include:
    A. airborne, droplet, and contact
    B. enteric, contact, and respiratory
    C. airborne, respiratory, and contact
    D. complete, droplet, and airborne

25. Which of the following is considered a fomite?
    A. phlebotomy tray
    B. handwashing
    C. immunizations
    D. transfusions

26. Which of the following isolation techniques requires that any blood collection equipment taken into the patient's room must be taken out after the blood is collected?
    A. droplet precautions
    B. reverse isolation
    C. contact precautions
    D. A and C

27. Disinfectants are:
    A. quaternary ammonium compounds
    B. chemicals that are used to inhibit the growth and development of microorganisms but do not necessarily kill them
    C. chemicals that are used to remove or kill pathogenic microorganisms
    D. used frequently on skin

28. A factor that increases a host's susceptibility in the chain of infection is:
    A. use of disposable equipment
    B. proper nutrition
    C. an immunization
    D. drug use

29. Contact precautions may be required for patients infected with:
    A. infectious tuberculosis
    B. herpes simplex
    C. rubella
    D. measles

30. Which of the following chemicals has the fastest speed of action in hand-hygiene antiseptic cleaning?
    A. iodophors
    B. phenol derivatives
    C. chlorhexidine
    D. 70% isopropyl alcohol

31. In health care facilities, which is a typical fomite?
    A. chlorhexidene
    B. hexachlorophene
    C. laboratory coat
    D. iodine for blood culture collections

32. The work status of a health care provider should be "off from work" if he or she has:
    A. chicken pox
    B. herpes simplex
    C. hepatitis C
    D. gonorrhea

33. Which of the following is the most important procedure in the prevention of disease transmission in health care institutions?
    A. reporting personal illnesses to supervisor
    B. use of appropriate waste disposal practices
    C. use of PPE
    D. hand hygiene

34. Which of the following would require droplet precautions?
   A. *Mycoplasma pneumonia*
   B. *Shigella*
   C. *Escherichia coli*
   D. *Clostridium difficile*

35. Which of the following is designed to reduce the risk of transmission of microorganisms from both recognized and unrecognized sources of infection in health care facilities?
   A. airborne precautions
   B. standard precautions
   C. droplet precautions
   D. wound isolation

36. Vectors in transmitting infectious diseases include:
   A. rabies
   B. *Salmonella*
   C. mites
   D. age

37. Which type of isolation precaution is frequently required for patients with infections that are transmitted through direct hand contact with colonized microorganisms?
   A. droplet precautions
   B. skin isolation
   C. reverse isolation
   D. contact precautions

38. Babies whose mothers have which of the following problems must be isolated from other infants?
   A. genital herpes
   B. kidney failure and are in a dialysis unit
   C. burns
   D. cancer

39. What infectious agent affecting a patient requires the use of a personal respirator by the phlebotomist?
   A. *Escherichia coli*
   B. *Mycobacterium tuberculosis*
   C. *Shigella*
   D. *Salmonella*

40. Which of the following is *not* a component that makes up the chain of infection?
   A. mode of transmission
   B. susceptible host
   C. mode of transportation
   D. source

41. If an accident occurs, such as a needlestick, the injured health care provider should immediately:
   A. contact his or her immediate supervisor
   B. fill out the necessary health care forms
   C. take the needle back to the clinical laboratory for verification of the accident
   D. cleanse the area with isopropyl alcohol and apply an adhesive bandage

42. To prevent skin and mucous membrane exposure when contact with a patient's blood is anticipated, which of the following should be worn?
   A. BBP
   B. PPE
   C. CDC
   D. FDA

43. Which of the following diseases usually require(s) airborne precautions?
   A. herpes simplex
   B. wound infections
   C. pertussis
   D. tuberculosis

44. When collecting blood from neonates in the nursery, what health-care-acquired infection is highly prevalent?
    A. rotavirus
    B. smallpox
    C. measles
    D. cholera

45. In Spanish, *peligro biologico* refers to the English term:
    A. hepatitis
    B. bloodborne pathogen
    C. *Salmonella*
    D. biohazardous

46. Therapeutic measures (i.e., chemotherapy, radiation therapy) in a patient create what part of the chain of infection?
    A. susceptible host
    B. source
    C. mode of transmission
    D. pathogen

47. Proper handwashing prior to and after blood collection requires rubbing wet, soapy hands together vigorously for at least:
    A. 5 seconds
    B. 15 seconds
    C. 45 seconds
    D. 1 minute

48. In addition to standard precautions, use contact precautions for patients with known:
    A. *Haemophilus influenzae*
    B. wound infections
    C. rubella
    D. mumps

49. Which of the following requires respiratory protective equipment for the phlebotomist?
    A. contact precautions
    B. airborne precautions
    C. droplet precautions
    D. standard precautions

50. Good nutrition can break the chain of nosocomial infections between the:
    A. source and the mode of transmission
    B. mode of transportation and the susceptible host
    C. source and the susceptible host
    D. mode of transmission and the susceptible host

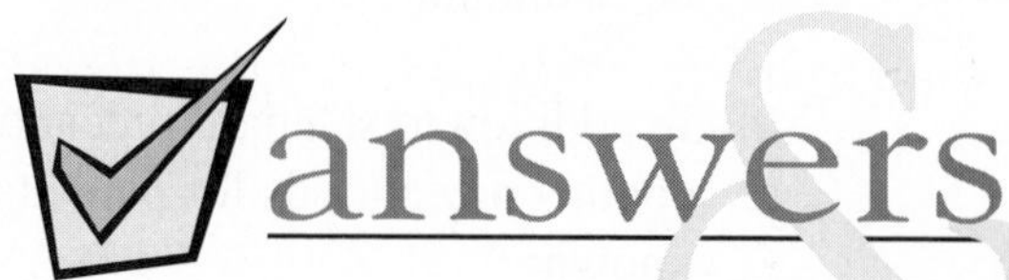

answers & rationales

1.

B. *Candida albicans* is a commonly identified pathogenic agent that causes health-care-acquired skin infections. (pp. 103–104)

2.

B. The clinical laboratory contributes to maintaining laboratory records for surveillance purposes, reporting on infectious agents and drug-resistant microorganisms, and evaluating the effectiveness of sterilization or decontamination procedures. It is *not* involved in decontaminating the surgery rooms with disinfectants. (p. 131)

3.

D. Transmission-based precautions to reduce the transmission of meningitis are referred to as droplet precautions. (p. 111)

4.

C. The last step after collecting blood in an isolation room is to wash your hands. (p. 128)

5.

B. An outbreak of particular health-care-acquired infections in a health care facility is detected through infection control surveillance. (p. 118)

6.

C. Health-care-acquired infections occur when the chain of infection is complete. (p. 109)

7.

C. Nosocomial (health-care-acquired) infections are those that are acquired by a patient after admission to a health care facility. (p. 102)

8.

A. *Escherichia coli* is a commonly identified pathogenic agent that causes nosocomial infections in the nursery unit. (p. 103)

9.

B. After gowning, a mask (if necessary) may be put over the nose and mouth. Then, gloves should be put on and pulled over the ends of gown sleeves. (pp. 124–125)

10.

D. Iodine solutions are commonly used to cleanse the skin for blood culture collections. (p. 132)

11.

D. The Joint Commission requires the development and implementation of an infection control program in a health care facility. (p. 102)

12.

C. The CDC, as part of the U.S. Public Health Service, oversees the investigation and control of various diseases. (p. 102)

13.

A. Nosocomial infections occur when the chain of infection is complete. The three components that make up the chain are the source, mode of transmission, and susceptible host. (p. 109)

14.

B. Alcohols and iodine compounds are most effective for *Mycobacterium tuberculosis.* (p. 133)

15.

B. *Vibrio cholerae* is a pathogenic agent that causes health-care-acquired infections of the gastrointestinal tract. (p. 104)

16.

C. The label shown in Figure 4.1 will most likely be posted in the entrance to the TB culture area since the label is a biohazardous sign and cautions against entering an area that can lead to an infection. (p. 106)

17.

A. Hexylresorcinol is an antiseptic for skin that is used frequently in surgery. (p. 132)

18.

D. Good nutrition interrupts the chain of nosocomial infection between the susceptible host and the source. (pp. 110–111)

19.

C. Reverse, or protective, isolation is used for patients who have immunodeficiency disorders to protect them from external environments. (p. 121)

20.

C. Of the 35 million patients admitted to hospitals annually in the United States, 1.75–3 million patients acquire a nosocomial infection. (p. 102)

21.

C. Diphtheria infection leads to droplet precautions due to coughing. (p. 113)

22.

B. Strep throat (group A) requires that the employee be placed on appropriate antibiotics for 24 hours before he or she may come to work. (p. 108)

23.

B. The warning label in Figure 4.2 was originally established as a requirement by OSHA. (p. 105)

24.

A. Under the most recent CDC isolation guidelines, three sets of precautions include airborne, droplet, and contact. (p. 111)

25.

A. Scrub suits, computer keyboards, phlebotomy trays, doorknobs, and telephones are a few examples of fomites (objects that can harbor infectious agents and transmit infections). (p. 110)

26.

D. Except for protective (reverse) isolation, any of the transmission-based precautions require that any articles contaminated with potentially infected material in the isolation room must be take out. (pp. 111–121)

27.

C. Disinfectants are chemical compounds that are used to remove or kill pathogenic microorganisms. (p. 132)

28.

D. Drug use is definitely a factor that affects a host's susceptibility to infection, since drug use decreases the status of the person's immune resistance. (p. 110)

29.

B. Contact precautions are used for herpes simplex. (p. 111)

30.

D. Alcohols (e.g., isopropyl alcohol) have the fastest speed of action for hand-hygiene antiseptic cleaning. (p. 133)

31.

C. Objects such as laboratory coats, eyeglasses, and computer keyboards that can harbor infectious agents and transmit infection are called fomites. (p. 110)

32.

A. For 7 days after the eruption of chicken pox, the employee should not work. (p. 108)

33.

D. Frequent hand hygiene is the most important procedure in the prevention of disease transmission in health care facilities. In any isolation procedures, it should be the first and last step. (pp. 103, 110, 116)

34.

A. *Mycoplasma pneumonia* requires droplet precautions. (pp. 113)

35.

B. Standard precautions are designed to reduce the risk of transmission of microorganisms from both recognized and unrecognized sources of infection in health care facilities. (p. 111)

36.

C. Mites act as vectors in transmitting infectious diseases. (pp. 109–110)

37.

D. Contact precautions prevent transmission of known or suspected infected or colonized microorganisms by direct hand or skin to skin contact for conditions such as in hepatitis A. (p.113)

38.

A. Babies whose mothers have genital herpes must be isolated from other infants. (p. 121)

39.

B. *Mycobacterium tuberculosis* causes a lung infection that can lead to airborne transmission to someone else. Thus, a personal respirator is required to be used by the health care worker when providing care to a patient with this infection. (pp. 113, 116)

40.

C. The three components that make up the chain are the source, mode of transmission, and susceptible host. (p. 109)

41.

D. If an accident occurs, such as a needlestick, the health care provider should immediately cleanse the area with isopropyl alcohol and apply a bandage. (p. 107)

42.

B. PPEs are barriers (i.e., gloves, facial masks, respirators, etc.) that should be worn to prevent skin and mucous membrane exposure when contact with a patient's blood is anticipated. (p. 115)

43.

D. A person with a tuberculosis infection would have airborne precautions to reduce the spread of airborne droplet transmission. (p. 113)

44.

A. Rotavirus is a highly prevalent health-care-acquired infection in the nursery unit of a health care facility. (p. 103)

45.

D. In Spanish, *peligro biologico* refers to the English term "biohazardous." (p. 105)

46.

A. Therapeutic measures (i.e., chemotherapy, radiation therapy) in a patient create the "susceptible host" in the chain of infection. (p. 110)

47.

B. Proper hand-washing, prior to and after blood collection, requires rubbing wet, soapy hands together vigorously for at least 15 seconds. (p. 117)

48.

B. Contact precautions are used for patients with wound infections. (p. 113)

49.

B. Respiratory protective equipment for the phlebotomist is required for airborne precautions. (p. 113)

50.

C. Good nutrition interrupts the chain of nosocomial infection between the source and the susceptible host. (pp. 110–111)

CHAPTER

5 Safety and First Aid

chapter objectives

Upon completion of Chapter 5, the learner is responsible for the following:

1. Discuss safety awareness for health care workers.
2. Explain the measures that should be taken for fire, electrical, radiation, mechanical, and chemical safety in a health care facility.
3. Describe the essential elements of a disaster emergency plan for a health care facility.
4. Explain the safety policies and procedures that must be followed in all phases of specimen collection and transportation.
5. Describe the safe use of equipment in health care facilities.
6. List three precautions that can reduce the risk of injury to patients.

DIRECTIONS Each of the questions or incomplete statements below is followed by four suggested answers or completions. Select one answer that is best in each case.

1. The label shown in Figure 5.1 will most likely be posted in the entrance to the:
   A. nursery
   B. nuclear medicine department
   C. TB culture area
   D. microbiology department

2. Chemicals should:
   A. be disposed of in the sink with water gently running
   B. be stored above eye level
   C. be cleaned in a spill with soap and water
   D. be labeled properly

3. If an electrical accident occurs involving electrical shock to an employee or a patient, the health care worker should first:
   A. shut off the electrical power source
   B. pull the electrocuted person from the electrical source
   C. call medical assistance and start cardiopulmonary resuscitation (CPR) immediately
   D. start CPR immediately

FIGURE 5.1

4. The abbreviation RACE is used in:
   A. radiation emergencies
   B. fire emergencies
   C. electrical emergencies
   D. mechanical emergencies

5. A dosimeter badge is required in health care facilities for:
   A. chemical safety
   B. fire safety
   C. radiation safety
   D. electrical safety

6. To be able to put out a fire safely, you should:
   A. know how to implement RACE
   B. locate where the dosimeter is located
   C. implement the (MSDS) system
   D. call the HazCom team

7. Class C fires involve:
   A. gasoline, paints, and/or oil
   B. electrical equipment
   C. wood and/or paper
   D. flammable materials

8. If acid gets on your skin, wash at once with:
   A. antimicrobial soap
   B. isopropyl alcohol
   C. water
   D. antimicrobial cleanser

9. Chemicals that are defined as explosive flammables must be stored:
   A. in a separate storage room
   B. in small carrying containers
   C. on a high shelf away from light and heat
   D. in an explosion-proof or fireproof room or cabinet

10. An MSDS is used for information on:
    A. patients
    B. phlebotomy technical procedures
    C. chemicals
    D. sharps disposal containers

11. The hazardous labeling system developed by the NFPA has the blue quadrant of the diamond to indicate a:
    A. flammability hazard
    B. health hazard
    C. instability hazard
    D. specific hazard

12. Which of the following is the appropriate response to a fire in the health care institution?
    A. Immediately take the elevator to leave the area.
    B. Shut off the electrical power.
    C. If caught in the fire, run to the exit.
    D. Use an ABC extinguisher if the fire is small.

13. What are the major principles of self-protection from radiation exposure?
    A. distance, combustibility, and shielding
    B. time, distance, and shielding
    C. anticorrosive, shielding, and distance
    D. combustibility, anticorrosive, and distance

14. MSDSs must be supplied to employees according to the:
    A. Hazard Communication Standard (29 CFR 1910.1200)
    B. EPA standards
    C. NFPA
    D. CDC

15. If a health care worker has a chemical spilled onto him or her, he or she should first:
    A. rub vigorously with one hand
    B. wait to see whether the chemical starts to burn the skin
    C. rinse the area with a neutral chemical
    D. rinse the area with water

16. A fire that occurs near electrical equipment is classified as what type of fire?
    A. Class A
    B. Class B
    C. Class C
    D. Class D

17. When mixing acid and water, you should:
    A. add water to acid
    B. add acid to water
    C. add equal amounts in a glass container
    D. add equal amounts in a plastic container

18. The HazCom standard requires chemical manufacturers to supply:
    A. fire blankets and fire extinguishers
    B. nonlatex medical equipment
    C. DOTs
    D. MSDSs

19. When a victim's breathing movement stops or his or her lips, tongue, or fingernails become blue, immediately start breathing aid with which of the following being the first step?
    A. Place the victim on his or her back.
    B. See if the victim is conscious by gently tapping his or her shoulders and speaking "Are you okay?"
    C. Place one hand on the victim's forehead, apply firm, backward pressure with the palm, and tilt the head back.
    D. Pinch the victim's nose shut with your fingers and, after taking a deep breath, seal your mouth over the victim's mouth with a barrier device and blow two rescue breaths.

20. The Right to Know law originated with:
    A. CLIA '88
    B. DOT
    C. OSHA
    D. CDC

21. MSDS is an abbreviation for:
    A. material serum data sheets
    B. material safety drug sheets
    C. material safety data sheets
    D. material serum drug sheets

22. Which of the following should *not* be done for a shock victim who seems to be semiconscious?
    A. Elevate the victim's legs so that the head is lower than the trunk of the body.
    B. Give fluids to the victim to maintain hydration.
    C. Call for emergency assistance.
    D. Keep the victim's airway passage open.

23. Which of the following is needed for cleanup of a chemical spill?
    A. chlorhexidine and isopropyl alcohol
    B. rubber gloves
    C. NIOSH TB respirator
    D. nonlatex gloves

24. If a health care worker has a chemical splashed into his or her eye(s), the first thing he or she should do is:
    A. wipe the eye(s) with a sterile gauze
    B. run to the emergency room
    C. immediately flush the eye(s) with water for 15 minutes
    D. call the supervisor within the specimen collection area

25. For Class A fires, what type of fire extinguishers can be used?
    A. carbon dioxide, dry chemical
    B. dry chemical, pressurized water
    C. halon, dry chemical
    D. carbon dioxide, halon

26. The chemicals with a blue storage code indicates that they
    A. are highly corrosive
    B. may detonate
    C. are a health hazard
    D. are flammable

27. In an emergency, a tourniquet should be used to control bleeding for:
    A. a cut that is bleeding on the lower arm
    B. an amputated leg or arm
    C. a leg that has a cut to the ankle area
    D. an arm that is lacerated above the elbow

28. Which of the following actions is followed for chemical safety in the health care facility?
    A. Chemicals should be stored at least above eye level for easy visibility.
    B. It is not advisable to use aprons in addition to laboratory coats for protection against chemicals.
    C. An acid carrier should be used when transporting alkalis or acids.
    D. Explosives that may create a fire should be stored only in an explosion-proof room.

29. Which of the following is the first step to take when finding someone who is severely bleeding?
    A. Immediately apply a tourniquet to the bleeding limb.
    B. Run for medical assistance.

C. Apply pressure directly over the wound.
D. Raise the injured limb above the level of the victim's heart.

30. When using a fire extinguisher, the operator should try to remember the acronym:
A. OSHA
B. PASS
C. RACE
D. CDC

31. CPR stands for cardiopulmonary:
A. rescue
B. resuscitation
C. return
D. recovery

32. According to the hazard labeling system developed by the NFPA, the yellow quadrant of the diamond indicates:
A. a flammability hazard
B. a health hazard
C. an instability hazard
D. a specific hazard

33. Which of the following is *not* reported as a warning through the NFPA?
A. fire
B. chemical instability
C. PPE
D. health hazard

34. The health care provider is most likely to encounter which of the following hazards upon entering the nuclear medicine department to obtain a blood specimen from a patient?
A. a fire hazard
B. a radiation hazard
C. a mechanical hazard
D. an electrical hazard

35. Which of the following actions is recommended if first aid is given to a shock victim?
A. Give fluids to the victim in order to keep him or her hydrated.
B. Place cold packs around the victim to slow his or her metabolism down, which will decrease further injury.
C. Keep the victim lying down.
D. Elevate the victim's head so that it is higher than the trunk of the body.

36. If a health care provider is caught in a fire in the health care institution, he or she should *not:*
A. run
B. close all the doors and windows before leaving the area
C. attempt to extinguish the fire if it is small
D. call the assigned fire number

37. MSDSs are used for:
A. mechanical safety
B. electrical safety
C. chemical safety
D. fire safety

38. The red quadrant of the NFPA rating system indicates what type of hazard?
A. health hazard
B. acid or alkali hazard
C. fire hazard
D. instability hazard

39. Safety equipment in the chemical area of the health care facility will most likely include:
A. dosimeter readers
B. an emergency shower
C. a mouth-to-mouth barrier device
D. respirator masks

40. If a fire extinguisher has to be used in a health care environment, the first step to perform is:
    A. squeeze the handle of the extinguisher to spray the solution on the fire
    B. pull the pin off the extinguisher
    C. spray the solution from the extinguisher towards the base of the fire
    D. aim the extinguisher at the gase of fire

41. Electrical safety involves:
    A. knowing the locations of fire extinguishers in the health care facility
    B. distance, time, and shielding
    C. knowing the location of the circuit breaker box
    D. knowing the MSDS codes

42. What organization developed a labeling system for hazardous chemicals that are frequently used in health care facilities?
    A. FDA
    B. NFPA
    C. CDC
    D. CLSI

43. Which of the following PPE can be used without precautionary evaluation when the phlebotomist must enter a latex-safe environment?
    A. gloves
    B. laboratory coat
    C. tourniquet
    D. syringe

44. High exposures of radioactivity have been shown to lead to:
    A. diabetes
    B. leukemia
    C. rheumatoid arthritis
    D. multiple sclerosis

45. To put out a fire in a person's hair or clothes, use
    A. the fire extinguisher for Class D fires
    B. a first-aid kit
    C. the fire extinguisher for Class C fires
    D. a fire blanket

46. The first step in giving mouth-to-mouth resuscitation is to:
    A. open the airway by checking for obstructions
    B. listen and feel for return of air from the victim's mouth
    C. determine whether the victim is conscious by gently shaking the victim and yelling, "Are you okay?"
    D. look for the victim's chest to rise and fall

47. To perform CPR on an individual, what primary equipment is required?
    A. face shield
    B. mouth-to-mouth barrier device
    C. gloves
    D. laboratory coat for personal protection

48. A bottle of sulfuric acid may be carried through the health care facility in
    A. your hand
    B. your latex-free gloved hand
    C. an acid carrier
    D. a heavy cardboard box

49. MSDSs list which of the following?
    A. EPA standards

B. emergency information, precautionary measures and phone numbers of local emergency shelters
C. NFPA standards
D. precautionary measures, general information on chemical and emergency information

50. If a health care provider is in an area of the health care facility where a fire starts, he or she should *first:*
A. attempt to extinguish the fire, using the proper equipment
B. pull the lever in the fire alarm box
C. close all the doors and windows before leaving the area
D. block the entrances so that others will not enter the fire area

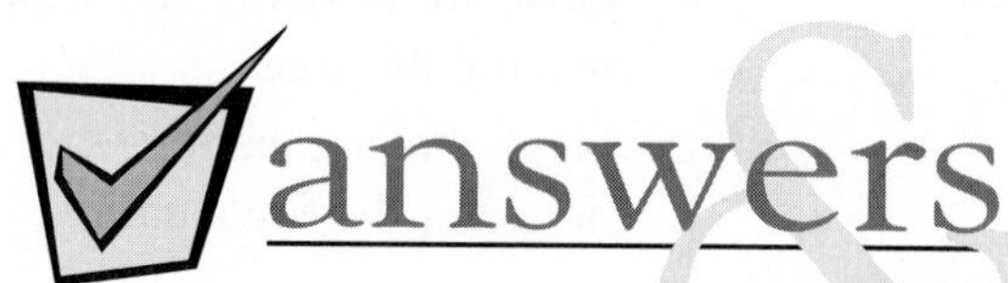

answers & rationales

1.

B. The label shown in Figure 5.1 will be posted at the entrance of the nuclear medicine department. (p. 143)

2.

D. All chemicals must be labeled properly since they pose health and/or physical hazards. (pp. 144–145)

3.

A. If an electrical accident has occurred involving electrical shock to an employee or a patient, the health care worker should shut off the electrical power and call for medical assistance and immediately start CPR. (p. 143)

4.

B. RACE is used in fire emergencies. (p. 141)

5.

C. A dosimeter badge is required in health care facilities for radiation safety. (p. 143)

6.

A. To be able to put out a fire safely, you should know how to implement RACE. (p. 141)

7.

B. Class C fires involve electrical equipment. (p. 140)

8.

C. If acid gets on your skin, rinse immediately with large amounts of water. (p. 147)

9.

D. Any explosive flammables must be stored in an explosion-proof or fireproof room or cabinet. (p. 146)

10.

C. MSDS is required for any chemicals with a hazard warning label. (pp. 144–145)

11.

B. The blue quadrant of the NFPA's 0–4 hazard rating system indicates a health hazard. (p. 146)

12.

D. The appropriate response to a fire in the health care institution is to use an ABC extinguisher if the fire is small. (pp. 141–142)

13.

B. The three cardinal principles of self-protection from radiation exposure are time, distance, and shielding. (p. 143)

14.

A. OSHA amended the Hazard Communication Standard (29 CFR 1910.1200) to include health care facilities. Thus labels for hazardous chemicals must (1) provide a warning (e.g., corrosive), (2) explain the nature of the hazard, (3) state special precautions to eliminate risks, and (4) explain first-aid treatment in the event of a leak, a chemical spill, or other exposure to the chemical. (pp. 144–145)

15.

D. The victim of a chemical accident must immediately rinse the affected area with water for at least 15 minutes after removing contaminated clothing. (p. 147)

16.

C. A fire that occurs in or near electrical equipment is a Class C fire. (p. 140)

17.

B. ALWAYS add acid to water. NEVER add water to acid. (p. 145)

18.

D. The HazCom standard requires chemical manufacturers to supply MSDSs. (pp. 144–145)

19.

B. When a victim's breathing movement stops or his or her lips, tongue, or fingernails become blue, immediately start breathing aid with the first step being seeing if the victim is conscious by gently tapping his or her shoulders and speaking "Are you okay?" (p. 152)

20.

C. The Right to Know law originated with OSHA. (p. 144)

21.

C. MSDS is an abbreviation for material safety data sheets. (pp. 144–145)

22.

B. A shock victim who is semiconscious should not be given fluids. (p. 154)

23.

B. For cleanup of a chemical spill, the health care worker should immediately obtain a spill cleanup kit that includes rubber gloves. (p. 147)

24.

C. If a health care worker has a chemical splashed into his or her eye(s), he or she should rinse his or her eye(s) at the eyewash station for a minimum of 15 minutes. (p. 147)

25.

B. For Class A fires, you can use dry chemical and/or pressurized water fire extinguishers. (p. 140)

26.

C. The chemicals with a blue storage code indicate they are a health hazard. (p. 146)

27.

B. A tourniquet should not be used to control bleeding in an emergency except in the case of an amputated, mangled, or crushed arm or leg or for profuse bleeding that cannot be stopped otherwise. (p. 151)

28.

C. An acid carrier should be used when transporting alkalis or acids. (p. 146)

29.

C. Severe bleeding from an open wound can be immediately controlled by applying pressure directly over the wound using Standard Precautions. (p. 151)

30.

B. When using a fire extinguisher, the operator should try to remember the acronym PASS for *P*ull pin; *A*im nozzle; *S*queeze handle; and *S*weep side to side. (p. 140)

31.

B. CPR stands for cardiopulmonary resuscitation. (pp. 151–152)

32.

C. The yellow quadrant of the NFPA's 0–4 hazard rating system indicates an instability hazard. (p. 146)

33.

C. The NFPA provides warning information for fires and a labeling system for hazardous chemicals, but does not oversee PPE. (pp. 145–146)

34.

B. The health care provider is most likely to encounter a radiation hazard when he or she enters the nuclear medicine department to obtain a blood specimen from a patient. (p. 143)

35.

C. The shock victim should be kept in a lying position. (p. 154)

36.

A. If a health care provider is caught in a fire in the health care institution, he or she should *not* run. (p. 141)

37.

C. MSDSs are used for chemical safety. (pp. 144–145)

38.

C. The red quadrant of the NFPA's 0–4 rating system indicates a fire hazard. (p. 146)

39.

B. Safety equipment maintained in the chemical area of the health care facility will most likely include an emergency shower. (p. 147)

40.

B. If a fire extinguisher has to be used in a health care environment, the first step to perform is pulling the pin off the extinguisher. (p. 141)

41.

C. Electrical safety in the health care facility involves knowing the location of the circuit breaker box. (p. 142)

42.

B. The NFPA developed a labeling system for hazardous chemicals that is frequently used in health care facilities. (pp. 145–146)

43.

B. A laboratory coat is a PPE that is not made of latex and can be used without latex precautions. (pp. 149–150)

44.

B. High exposures of radioactivity have been shown to lead to leukemia. (p. 143)

45.

D. The fire blanket should be used to smother a person's burning clothes, hair, etc. (p. 139)

46.

C. The first step in giving mouth-to-mouth resuscitation is to determine whether the victim is conscious by gently shaking the victim and yelling, "Are you okay?" (p. 152)

47.

B. To perform CPR on an individual, the primary equipment required is a mouth-to-mouth barrier device. (p. 152)

48.

C. A bottle of sulfuric acid may be carried through the health care facility in an acid carrier. (p. 146)

49.

D. MSDSs list precautionary measures, general information on chemical and emergency information. (p. 145)

50.

B. If a health care provider is in an area of the health care facility where a fire starts, he or she should *first* pull the lever in the fire alarm box. (p. 141)

CHAPTER

6 Medical Terminology, Anatomy, and Physiology of Organ Systems

chapter objectives

Upon completion of Chapter 6, the learner is responsible for the following:

1. Define medical terminology using word elements such as roots, prefixes, and suffixes.
2. Define words commonly used in the clinical laboratory.
3. Describe how laboratory testing is used to assess body functions and disease.
4. Define the differences among the terms *anatomy, physiology,* and *pathology.*
5. Describe the directional terms, anatomic surface regions, and cavities of the body.
6. Describe the role of homeostasis in normal body functioning.
7. Describe the purpose, function, and structural components of the major body systems.
8. Identify examples of pathologic conditions associated with each organ system.

9. Describe the types of specimens that are analyzed in the clinical laboratory.
10. List common diagnostic tests associated with each organ system.

DIRECTIONS Each of the questions or incomplete statements below is followed by four suggested answers or completions. Select one answer that is best in each case.

1. A prefix is which of the following?
   A. the main part of a word
   B. a word element added after a word root
   C. a word element added before a word root
   D. a vowel that changes the word meaning

2. Upper extremities include which regions of the body?
   A. ankle and foot
   B. leg
   C. hand and wrist
   D. pelvis

3. The human torso usually refers to which of the following regions of the body?
   A. leg and foot
   B. arm and wrist
   C. face
   D. thorax, abdomen, and pelvis

4. The suffix that can be used to mean "tumor" is which of the following?
   A. osis
   B. philia
   C. oma
   D. plasia

5. The suffix that can be used to mean "cell" is which of the following?
   A. cyte
   B. logy
   C. scopy
   D. poiesis

6. The suffix that can be used to mean "the study of" is which of the following?
   A. cyte
   B. logy
   C. scopy
   D. poiesis

7. The root word that can be used to mean "clot" is which of the following?
   A. thromb
   B. veni
   C. derm
   D. arterio

8. The root word that can be used to mean "heart" is which of the following?
   A. cardi
   B. veni
   C. phleb
   D. embol

9. The root word that can be used to mean "pulse" is which of the following?
   A. capillus
   B. arterio
   C. pulmonary
   D. sphygmo

For que

10. The prefix that can be used to mean "small" is which of the following?
    A. centi
    B. micro
    C. mega
    D. uni

11. The prefix that can be used to mean "around" is which of the following?
    A. ante
    B. ambi
    C. peri
    D. poly

12. The prefix that can be used to mean "false" is which of the following?
    A. pseudo
    B. nulli
    C. infra
    D. retro

13. The term "gynecology" refers to which of the following?
    A. microscopic structures of bacteria
    B. study of female reproductive system
    C. urinary system structures
    D. bones and joints

14. The term "hepatitis" refers to which of the following?
    A. gall bladder rupture
    B. broken bone in the hip
    C. inflammation of the liver
    D. radioactive cells in the blood

15. The term "peritonitis" refers to which of the following?
    A. colon obstruction
    B. inflammation of the abdominal wall
    C. inflammation of the nasal membranes
    D. gas in the pancreas and stomach

16. The term that relates to the study of antibodies in the serum is which of the following?
    A. hematology
    B. histology
    C. anesthesiology
    D. immunology

17. The term that relates to the study of blood and blood-forming tissues is which of the following?
    A. histology
    B. cardiology
    C. oncology
    D. hematology

18. The term that relates to an inflammation of the skin is which of the following?
    A. dermatitis
    B. meningitis
    C. hepatitis
    D. osteomyelitis

19. The lumbar region refers to which of the following?
    A. larynx
    B. chest
    C. lower back
    D. head and neck

20. The axillary region refers to which of the following?
    A. armpit
    B. knee
    C. neck
    D. elbow

25. Which side of the body is represented by the directional arrow labeled “1” on the backside of the figure?
    A. medial
    B. cranial
    C. dorsal
    D. midlateral

26. Which plane of the body is represented by “2”?
    A. medial
    B. frontal/coronal
    C. transverse/horizontal
    D. midlateral

27. Which side of the body is represented by the directional arrow labeled “3”?
    A. dorsal/posterior
    B. cranial/cephalic/superior
    C. pericardial
    D. thoracic

28. Which plane of the body is represented by “4”?
    A. medial
    B. frontal/coronal
    C. transverse/horizontal
    D. midlateral

29. Which side of the body is represented by the directional arrow labeled “5”?
    A. dorsal/posterior
    B. cranial/cephalic/superior
    C. medial
    D. lateral

30. Which side of the body is represented by the directional arrow labeled “6”?
    A. dorsal/posterior
    B. cranial/cephalic/superior
    C. medial
    D. lateral

31. What is the most likely organ represented by “7”?
    A. shoulder blade
    B. lung
    C. armpit
    D. gall bladder

32. What is the most likely organ represented by “8”?
    A. trachea
    B. lung
    C. alveoli
    D. bronchi

For questions 33–35, refer to Figure 6.3

FIGURE 6.3

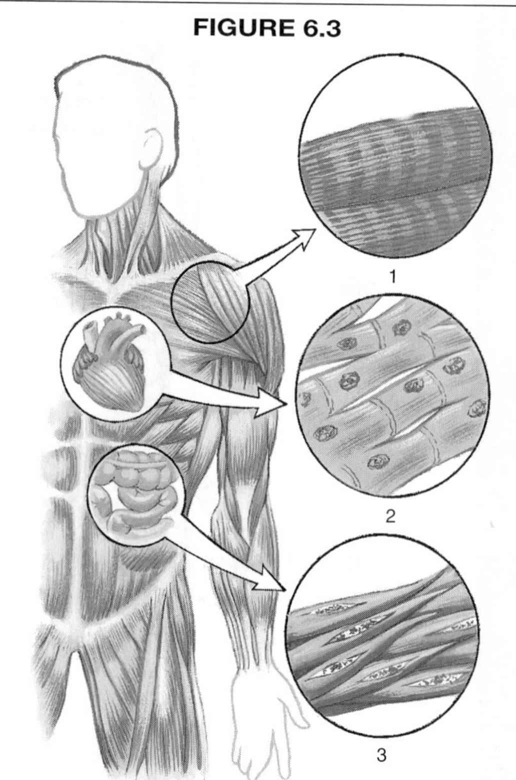

33. What type of muscle is represented by "1"?
  A. smooth
  B. tendons
  C. cardiac
  D. skeletal

34. What type of muscle is represented by "2"?
  A. smooth
  B. tendons
  C. cardiac
  D. skeletal

35. What type of muscle is represented by "3"?
  A. smooth
  B. tendons
  C. cardiac
  D. skeletal

For questions 36–38, refer to Figure 6.4 and answer questions about the shaded areas.

FIGURE 6.4

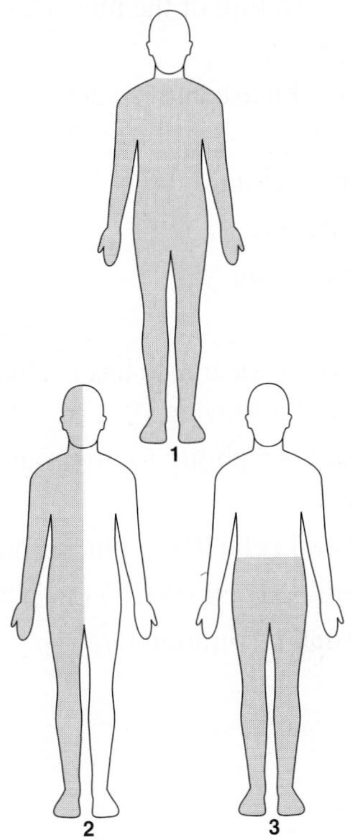

36. The shaded areas labeled "1" represent which type of paralytic condition?
  A. myalgia
  B. paraplegia
  C. hemiplegia
  D. quadriplegia

37. The shaded areas labeled "2" represent which type of paralytic condition?
  A. myalgia
  B. paraplegia
  C. hemiplegia
  D. quadriplegia

38. The shaded areas labeled "3" represent which type of paralytic condition?
  A. myalgia
  B. paraplegia
  C. hemiplegia
  D. quadriplegia

39. The proximal end of the forearm refers to which of the following?
  A. near the elbow
  B. around the fingers
  C. near the wrist
  D. by the shoulder

40. When speaking with a patient about which arm to use for a venipuncture, how should a phlebotomist refer to the right or left one?
  A. Refer to the phlebotomist's right/left side.
  B. Refer to the patient's right/left arm.
  C. Face the same way the patient is facing and point to the arm.
  D. Don't talk about it; just proceed with the arm that looks the best.

41. Homeostasis refers to:
    A. blood clotting
    B. a chemical imbalance
    C. an anabolism
    D. a steady-state condition

42. Which of the following body systems provides carbon dioxide and oxygen exchange?
    A. muscular
    B. respiratory
    C. reproductive
    D. nervous

43. Which of the following body systems is the primary regulator of hormones?
    A. digestive
    B. integumentary
    C. urinary
    D. endocrine

44. What are vital signs?
    A. excess water in lungs
    B. overheated body temperature
    C. excessive respiration and pulse
    D. temperature, pulse, blood pressure, and respiration rate

45. Meninges are defined as:
    A. control nerves
    B. causative agent of meningitis
    C. control reflexes
    D. protective membrane layers

46. The endocrine system can best be evaluated by:
    A. tissue biopsy
    B. testing spinal fluid
    C. blood gas analyses
    D. analyzing hormone levels

47. After oxygen crosses the respiratory membranes (in the lung) into the blood, about 97% of it combines with:
    A. carbon dioxide
    B. the iron-containing portion of hemoglobin
    C. carbaminohemoglobin
    D. hypochloride

48. What is the blood pH range of a normal body?
    A. 7.5 to 8.0
    B. 7.35 to 7.45
    C. 0 to 7
    D. 6.5 to 10

49. Laboratory testing of the muscular system would include:
    A. creatine kinase and lactate dehydrogenase
    B. serum calcium
    C. urine culture
    D. synovial fluid

50. The creatinine clearance test evaluates which of the following?
    A. the kidneys' ability to filter out waste products
    B. red blood cell (RBC) functioning
    C. white blood cell (WBC) morphology
    D. abnormal respiration rate

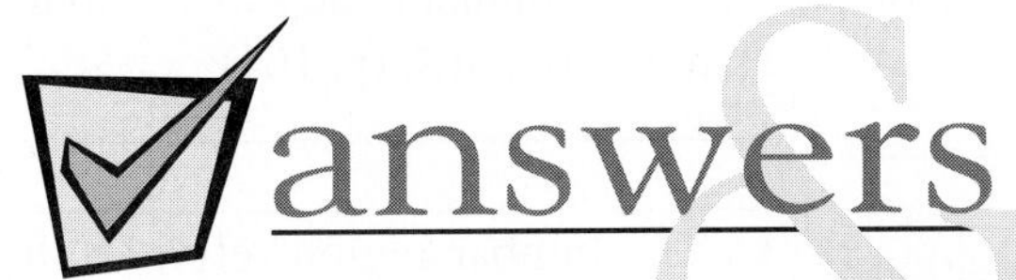

answers & rationales

1.

C. A prefix is a word element that is added before the root, at the beginning of the word. (p. 159)

2.

C. Upper extremities include arms and forearms, including the hand and wrist. (p. 168)

3.

D. The human torso refers to the trunk of the body, or the thorax, abdomen, and pelvis. (p. 168)

4.

C. The suffix that can be used to mean "tumor" is –oma, as in carcinoma. (p. 163)

5.

A. The suffix that can be used to mean "cell" is –cyte, as in lymphocyte. (p. 163)

6.

B. The suffix that can be used to mean "the study of" is –logy, as in cardiology. (p. 163)

7.

A. The root word that can be used to mean "clot" is thromb, as in thrombosis. (p. 162)

8.

A. The root word that can be used to mean "heart" is cardi/o, as in cardiology. (p. 162)

9.

D. The root word that can be used to mean "pulse" is sphygmo, as in sphygmomanometer. (p. 162)

10.

B. The prefix that can be used to mean "small" is micro, as in microscopic. (p. 161)

11.

C. The prefix that can be used to mean "around" is peri, as in periscope. (p. 161)

12.

A. The prefix that can be used to mean "false" is pseudo, as in pseudofracture. (p. 161)

13.

B. The term "gynecology" refers to the study of the female reproductive system. (p. 164)

14.

C. The term "hepatitis" refers to an inflammation of the liver. (p. 164)

15.

B. The term "peritonitis" refers to an inflammation of the abdominal wall. (p. 164)

16.

D. The term that relates to the study of antibodies in the serum is immunology. (p. 164)

17.

D. The term that relates to the study of blood and blood-forming tissues is hematology. (p. 164)

18.

A. The term that relates to an inflammation of the skin is dermatitis. (p. 164)

19.

C. The lumbar region refers to the lower back. (p. 172)

20.

A. The axillary region refers to the armpit area. (p. 172)

21.

B. Refer to Figure 6.5. (p. 169)

22.

D. Refer to Figure 6.5. (p. 169)

23.

C. Refer to Figure 6.5. (p. 169)

FIGURE 6.5

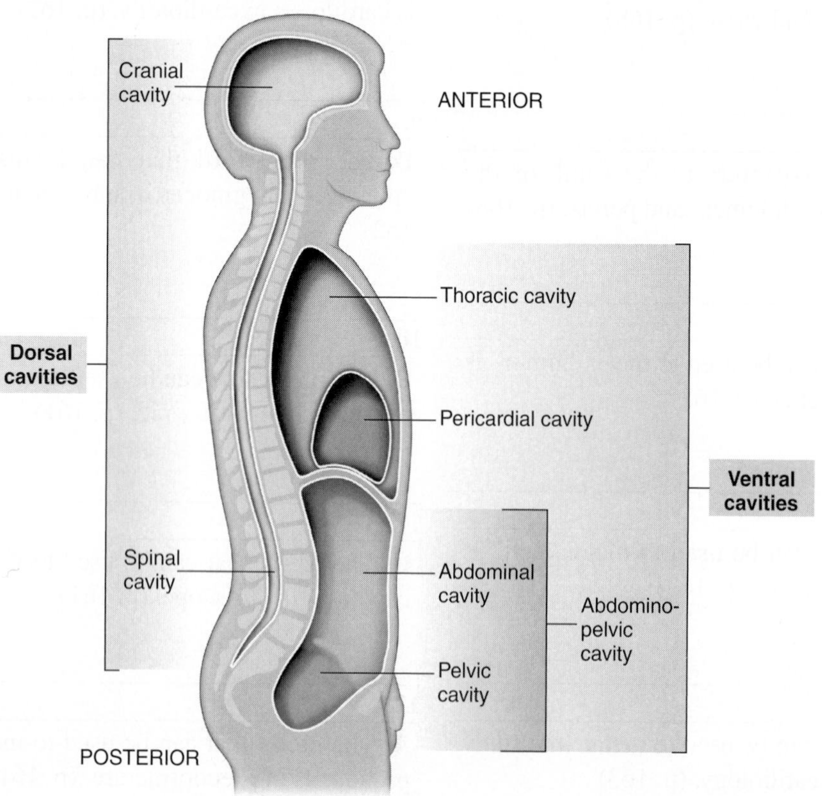

24.

A. Refer to Figure 6.5. (p. 169)

FIGURE 6.6

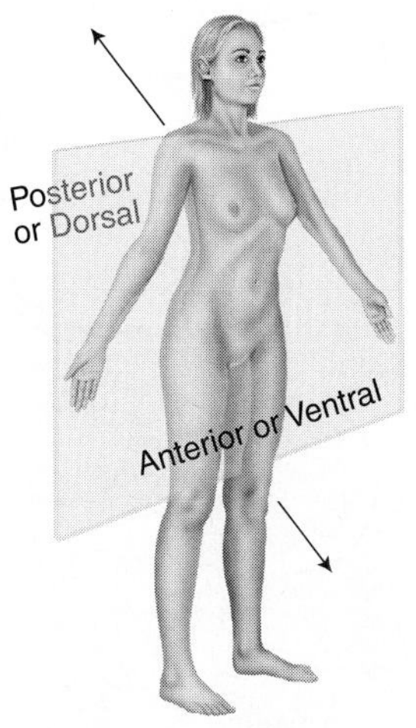

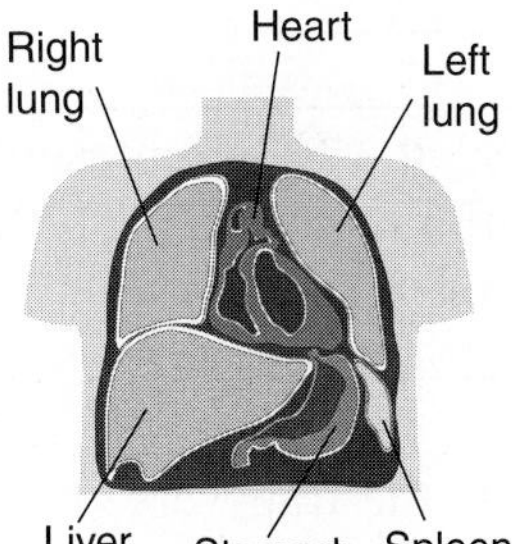

A Coronal (frontal) plane

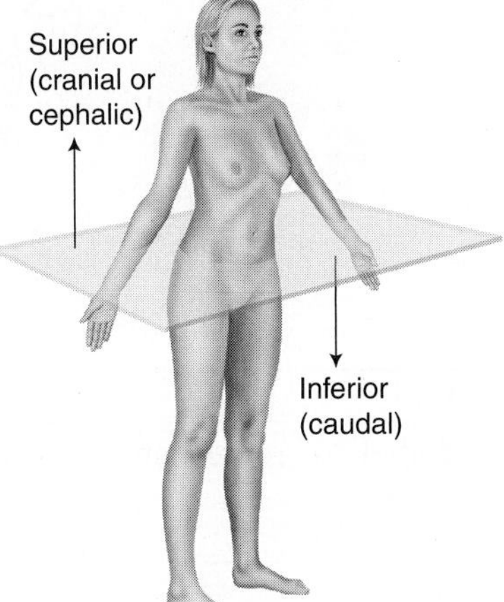

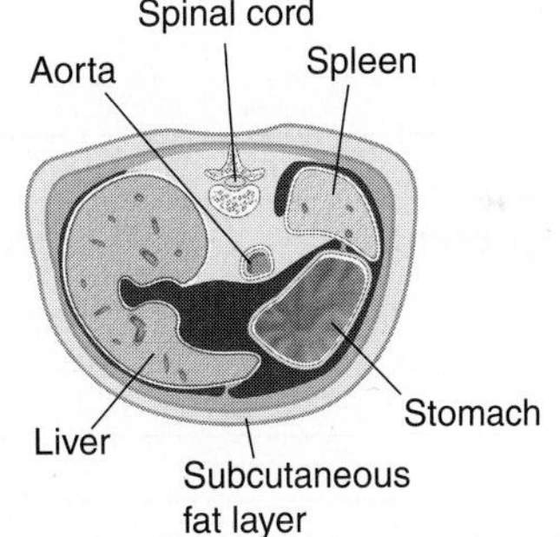

B Transverse (horizontal) plane

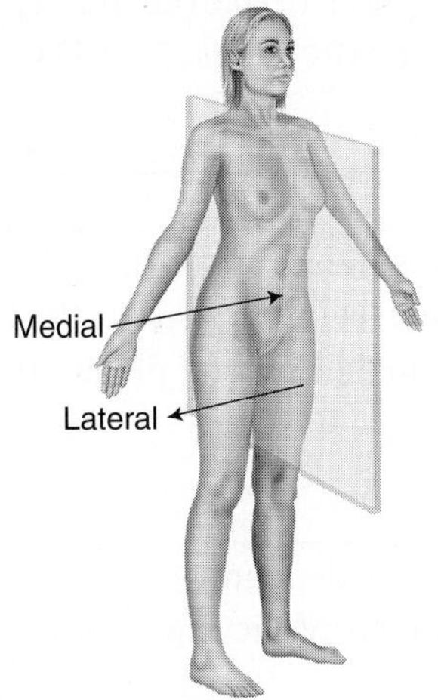

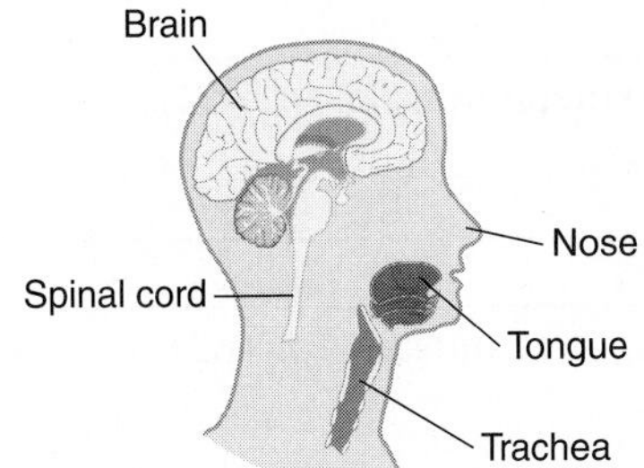

C Midsagittal (median) plane

25.

C. The arrow labeled "1" is the dorsal side. (p. 170)

26.

B. The "2" represents the frontal/coronal plane. (p. 170)

27.

B. The arrow labeled "3" represents the cranial/cephalic/superior direction. (p. 170)

28.

C. The "4" represents the transverse/horizontal plane. (p. 170)

29.

C. The "5" represents the medial direction. (p. 170)

30.

D. The "6" represents the lateral direction. (p. 170)

31.

B. The organ labeled "7" is the right lung. (p. 170)

32.

A. The part of the body labeled "8" is the trachea. (p. 170)

33.

Label "1" represents skeletal muscle. (p. 182)

34.

Label "2" represents cardiac muscle. (p. 182)

FIGURE 6.7

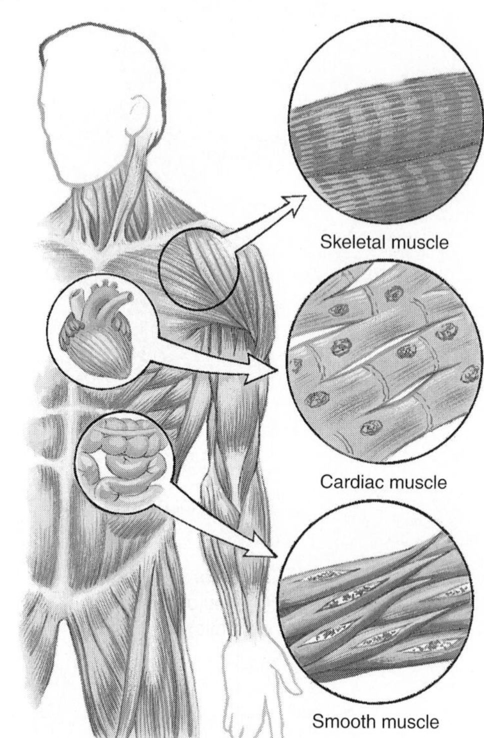

35.

Label "3" represents smooth muscle. (p. 182)

36.

The shaded areas in "1" represent quadriplegia, a complete or partial paralysis of the upper and lower extremities. (p. 187)

37.

The shaded areas in "2" represent hemiplegia, paralysis of one-half of the body when divided by the medial sagittal plane. (p. 187)

38.

The shaded areas in "3" represent paraplegia, paralysis of the lower part of the body. (p. 187)

FIGURE 6.8

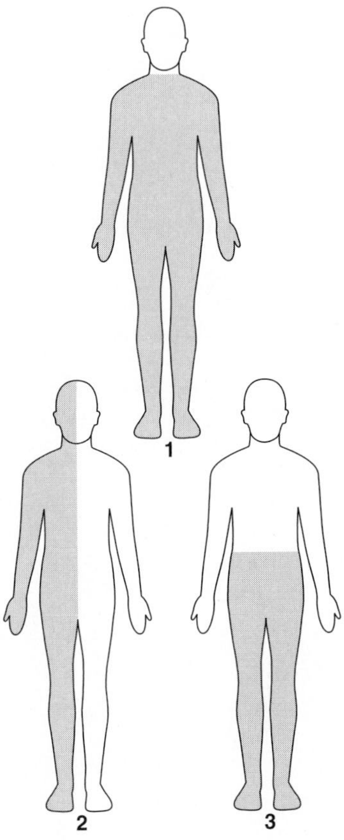

39.

The proximal end of the forearm refers to the end close to the point of attachment; in this case, it would be near the elbow. (p. 168)

40.

Phlebotomists should become accustomed to referring to the patient's right and left sides. It can be confusing when the phlebotomist is face-to-face with the patient. (p. 171)

41.

Homeostasis refers to a steady-state or chemically balanced condition in the body. (p. 166)

42.

The respiratory system allows carbon dioxide and oxygen exchange in the lungs. (pp. 188–189)

43.

The endocrine system is the primary regulator of hormones. (pp. 196–197)

44.

Vital signs are temperature, pulse, blood pressure, and respiration rate. (p. 167)

45.

Meninges are protective membranes around the brain and spinal cord. Between these membranes is cerebrospinal fluid (CSF) is also protective in nature. Phlebotomists are often responsible for transporting CSF to the laboratory for analysis. (p. 184)

46.

Since the endocrine system regulates hormone production, laboratory analysis of hormone levels is one way to evaluate this system. (pp. 197–198)

47.

Oxygen combines with the iron-containing portion of the hemoglobin molecule inside the RBCs. (pp. 188–189)

48.

Normal body pH has a narrow range of between 7.35 and 7.45. Deviations from the normal or reference range can be very dangerous to the patient. (p. 189)

49.

Laboratory testing of the muscular system could include assays of specific muscle enzymes such as creatine kinase and lactate dehydrogenase. (pp. 182–184)

50.

The creatinine clearance test evaluates the degree to which kidneys are filtering out waste products of metabolism. (pp. 193–195)

CHAPTER

7 The Cardiovascular and Lymphatic Systems

chapter objectives

Upon completion of Chapter 7, the learner is responsible for the following:

1. Define the functions of the cardiovascular and lymphatic systems.
2. Identify and describe the structures and functions of the heart.
3. List pathologic conditions and common laboratory tests associated with the cardiovascular and lymphatic systems.
4. Trace the flow of blood through the cardiovascular system.
5. Describe the properties of arterial blood, venous blood, and capillary blood.
6. Identify and describe the cellular and noncellular components of blood.
7. Describe the differences and similarities between whole blood, serum, and plasma.
8. Identify and describe the structures and functions of different types of blood vessels.

9. Locate and name the veins most commonly used for phlebotomy procedures.

10. Define hemostasis and describe the basic process of coagulation and fibrinolysis.

DIRECTIONS

Each of the questions or incomplete statements below is followed by four suggested answers or completions. Select one answer that is best in each case.

1. Which of the following is *not* a function of the cardiovascular system?
   A. storage of minerals for later use
   B. transportation of water and nutrients
   C. transportation of gases
   D. coagulation process

2. The term "systole" refers to:
   A. capillary dilation
   B. heart contraction
   C. heart relaxation
   D. pulmonary gas exchange

3. The term "diastole" refers to:
   A. capillary dilation
   B. heart contraction
   C. heart relaxation
   D. pulmonary gas exchange

4. In what location of the body does oxygen and carbon dioxide gas exchange take place?
   A. alveoli of the lungs
   B. heart
   C. arteries
   D. veins

5. How many times does the average normal adult heart beat each minute?
   A. 15–20
   B. 25–30
   C. 40–55
   D. 60–80

6. The term "leukocytes" is another name for:
   A. RBCs
   B. WBCs
   C. platelets
   D. sera

7. The term "erythrocytes" is another name for:
   A. RBCs
   B. WBCs
   C. platelets
   D. sera

8. The term "thrombocytes" is another name for:
   A. RBCs
   B. WBCs
   C. platelets
   D. sera

9. Serum is the liquid portion of a blood sample that:
   A. is highly oxygenated
   B. contains anticoagulant
   C. does not contain anticoagulant
   D. is rich in carbon monoxide

10. Plasma refers to a blood specimen that:
   A. is highly oxygenated
   B. contains fibrinogen
   C. does not contain anticoagulant
   D. is rich in carbon monoxide

11. Capillaries have which of the following characteristics?
    A. transport deoxygenated blood toward the heart
    B. transport oxygenated blood away from the heart
    C. link arterioles and venules
    D. carry only WBCs

12. Arteries have which of the following characteristics?
    A. transport deoxygenated blood toward the heart
    B. transport oxygenated blood away from the heart
    C. link arterioles and venules
    D. carry only RBCs

13. Veins have which of the following characteristics?
    A. transport deoxygenated blood toward the heart
    B. transport oxygenated blood away from the heart
    C. link arterioles and venules
    D. carry only RBCs

14. Which of the following reflects the primary function of leukocytes?
    A. oxygen transport
    B. host cells
    C. blood clotting
    D. defense against infections

15. Which of the following reflects the primary function of erythrocytes?
    A. oxygen transport
    B. host cells
    C. blood clotting
    D. defense against infections

16. Which of the following reflects the primary function of platelets?
    A. oxygen transport
    B. host cells
    C. blood clotting
    D. defense against infections

17. The process of blood cell development (hematopoiesis) includes which of the following?
    A. Cells begin as undifferentiated stem cells.
    B. It occurs every 200 days.
    C. It occurs in the lungs.
    D. It requires large volumes of water.

18. Which of the following features does *not* characterize RBCs?
    A. RBCs are biconcave disks that measure about 7 μm in diameter.
    B. They have no nuclei when circulating in the peripheral blood.
    C. They have a life span of about 120 days.
    D. They are smaller and more compact than platelets.

19. The upper chambers of the heart are the:
    A. right and left atria
    B. right and left ventricles
    C. inferior and superior vena cavae
    D. reticulocytes

20. The four chambers of the heart include the:
    A. right and left atria and ventricles
    B. four sided ventricles
    C. four sided atria
    D. superior and inferior chambers

21. Which statement describes plasma?
    A. It results when cellular components form a fibrin clot.
    B. It is normally bright or fluorescent yellow to orange.
    C. It is the fluid portion of unclotted blood.
    D. It contains only leukocytes.

22. Which statement describes serum?
    A. It results when cellular components form a fibrin clot.
    B. It is normally bright or fluorescent yellow to orange.
    C. It contains anticoagulant.
    D. It contains only leukocytes.

23. What happens to blood cells when a blood specimen is centrifuged?
    A. The cells lyse.
    B. The cells sink to the bottom of the tube.
    C. The cells and fluid are thoroughly mixed.
    D. Nothing happens to the specimen.

24. What is a thrombus?
    A. a leak in the vein
    B. heart attack
    C. a vessel wall
    D. a blood clot

25. What is arteriosclerosis?
    A. arthritis of the arteries
    B. thickening of the artery wall due to cholesterol
    C. blood clots within the vessels
    D. aortic stenosis

26. How is the heart rate measured?
    A. counting respirations per minute
    B. measuring oxygen content
    C. estimating blood volume
    D. taking the pulse rate

27. What is the most common blood type?
    A. A
    B. B
    C. AB
    D. O

28. What happens if a patient receives the wrong blood transfusion?
    A. Nothing abnormal happens to the patient.
    B. Transfusion reactions can lead to death.
    C. White cells begin to multiply abnormally.
    D. Nerve cells contract and cause pain.

29. A differential count refers to:
    A. blood pressure
    B. the contraction of the heart
    C. the enumeration of specific types of WBCs
    D. a heart murmur

30. Which arteries supply blood to the head and neck regions?
    A. hepatic
    B. subclavian
    C. brachial
    D. carotid

31. Which of the following is the major artery in the antecubital area of the arm?
    A. brachial
    B. carotid
    C. radial
    D. aorta

32. Which of the following veins is most commonly used for venipuncture?
    A. median cubital
    B. femoral
    C. great saphenous
    D. jugular

33. The term "buffy coat" refers to:
    A. erythrocytes and platelets
    B. leukocytes and platelets
    C. mononuclear cells
    D. protein and mineral deposits

34. A phlebotomist enters a room and the patient states that he or she is being treated with Coumadin. What does this mean for the phlebotomist?
    A. The patient's blood may clot slowly.
    B. The patient is diabetic and pregnant.
    C. The blood cell count is abnormally high.
    D. The phlebotomist should refer the patient to his or her doctor.

35. Which of the following best describes the term "hemostasis"?
    A. maintenance/retention of circulating blood in the vascular system
    B. vasoconstriction to prevent blood loss
    C. a steady-state condition
    D. clot retraction

36. The term "fibrinolysis" refers to:
    A. clot retraction
    B. platelet degranulation
    C. vasoconstriction
    D. dissolution of clot and regeneration of vessel

37. Tests for blood typing and cross-matching for donor blood are done in which of the following areas of the laboratory?
    A. hematology
    B. immunohematology
    C. clinical chemistry
    D. molecular pathology

38. Which of the following represents a reference range for a platelet count?
    A. $50,000/mm^3$
    B. $50,000–90,000/mm^3$
    C. $95,000–100,000/mm^3$
    D. $250,000–500,000/mm^3$

39. Which of the following statements best characterizes hemophilia?
    A. fear of needles
    B. fear of the sight of blood
    C. disease caused by internal blood clots
    D. excessive bleeding due to inadequate clotting factors

40. The longest vein in the body is the:
    A. saphenous
    B. median cubital
    C. aorta
    D. superior vena cava

41. How are bone marrow samples taken?
    A. aortic puncture
    B. aspiration from the iliac crest of the hip
    C. heel puncture
    D. subclavian puncture

42. Which one of the following is one reason why coagulation tests are ordered?
    A. presurgical workup
    B. to detect sickle cell anemia
    C. to detect congestive heart failure
    D. to diagnose leukemia or lymphoma

43. Platelet functions are assessed in the laboratory using:
    A. anticoagulated venous blood
    B. coagulated venous blood
    C. bone marrow aspirates
    D. capillary blood only from a finger puncture

FIGURE 7.1

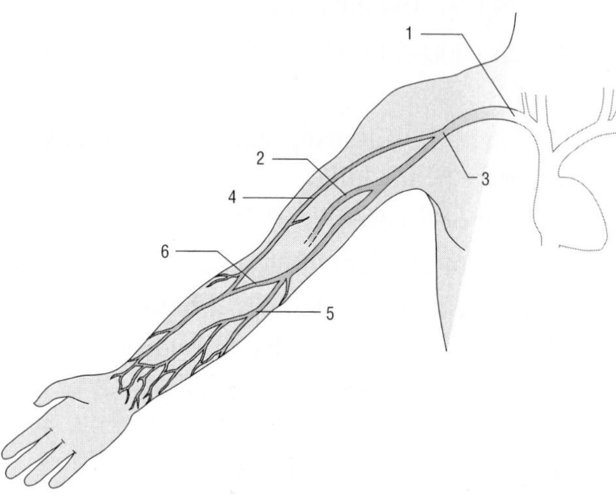

44. Hemoglobin content is assessed in the laboratory by analyzing:
    A. WBCs
    B. erythrocytes
    C. megakaryocytes
    D. platelets

For Questions 45–50, refer to Figure 7.1.

45. The vein labeled "1" most closely resembles which of the following veins?
    A. subclavian
    B. axillary
    C. cephalic
    D. basilic

46. The vein labeled "2" most closely resembles which of the following veins?
    A. subclavian
    B. axillary
    C. cephalic
    D. brachial

47. The vein labeled "3" most closely resembles which of the following veins?
    A. subclavian
    B. axillary
    C. cephalic
    D. basilic

48. The vein labeled "4" most closely resembles which of the following veins?
    A. subclavian
    B. axillary
    C. cephalic
    D. basilic

49. The vein labeled "5" most closely resembles which of the following veins?
    A. subclavian
    B. axillary
    C. cephalic
    D. basilic

50. The vein labeled "6" most closely resembles which of the following veins?
    A. median cubital
    B. axillary
    C. cephalic
    D. basilic

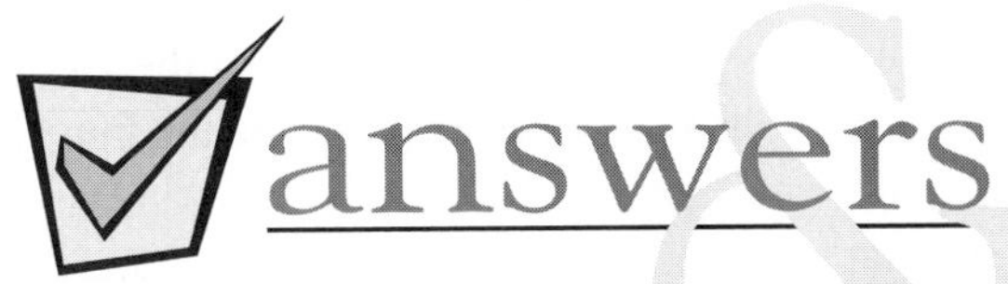

answers & rationales

1.

A. The cardiovascular system has main functions including transporting water and nutrients, transporting gases, regulating temperature, helping eliminate waste products, maintaining electrolyte balance, regulating the blood clotting system, and helping with immunity. However, the cardiovascular system does not store minerals for later use in the body; the skeletal system does this function. (p. 208)

2.

B. The term "systole" refers to heart muscle contraction. (p. 213)

3.

C. The term "diastole" refers to heart muscle relaxation. (p. 213)

4.

A. Oxygen and carbon dioxide gas exchange takes place in the alveoli of the lungs. (p. 211)

5.

D. The average normal adult heart beats 60–80 beats per minute. (p. 213)

6.

B. Leukocytes are white blood cells (WBCs). WBCs are divided further into cell lines that differ in color, size, shape, and nuclear formation. Leukocytes function primarily as part of the body's defense mechanism. (p. 221)

7.

A. Erythrocytes are red blood cells (RBCs). Approximately 99% of the circulating cells in the bloodstream are erythrocytes. They are biconcave disks that normally measure about 6–7 μm in diameter. Millions of hemoglobin molecules that function to carry oxygen to all parts of the body are present within each mature RBC. (pp. 222–224)

8.

C. Thrombocytes are platelets. Platelets are much smaller in size than the other circulating cells in the bloodstream. Normally, there are 250,000–500,000 platelets/mm^3. Platelets help initiate the blood clotting process. (pp. 222, 227)

9.

C. Serum is the liquid portion of the blood that remains after a blood specimen has been allowed to clot, and then centrifuged. Blood cells remain meshed in a fibrin clot. Serum does not contain anticoagulant. (pp. 223, 232–233)

10.

B. Plasma refers to a blood specimen that contains fibrinogen (AND an anticoagulant, a chemical substance that prevents blood from clotting. A blood specimen that has been anticoagulated can be separated by centrifugation into plasma and blood cells, but it has no fibrin clot. (pp. 223, 232–233)

11.

C. Capillaries are microscopic vessels that link arterioles to venules. They may be so small in diameter as to allow only one blood cell to pass through at any given time. Gas exchange occurs in the capillaries of tissues. (pp. 217–218)

12.

B. Arteries are vessels that carry highly oxygenated blood away from the heart. They branch into smaller vessels called arterioles and into capillaries. They normally have thicker walls, and a pulse. (pp. 216–218)

13.

A. Veins carry blood toward the heart. Because the blood in veins flows against gravity in many areas of the body, these vessels have one-way valves to prevent backflow and rely on muscular action to move blood cells through the vessels. All veins, except the pulmonary veins, contain deoxygenated blood and have thinner walls than arteries. The forearm vein that is most commonly used for venipuncture is the median cubital vein. (pp. 215–217)

14.

D. The primary function of leukocytes is defense. The cells phagocytize (ingest) pathogenic microorganisms and play a role in immunity through antibody production. (pp. 221–224)

15.

A. Erythrocytes function primarily to transport oxygen from the lungs to the tissues and carbon dioxide from the tissues to the lungs. (pp. 224–225)

16.

C. Platelets function in the blood clotting process. (pp. 227–228)

17.

A. Blood cells develop from undifferentiated stem cells in the hematopoietic or blood-forming tissues such as the bone marrow. Stem cells are considered immature because they have not yet developed into their functional state. The cells will undergo changes in their nucleus and cytoplasm so that they differentiate and become functional once they are in the circulating blood. (p. 221)

18.

D. RBCs are not smaller or more compact than platelets. (pp. 224–225)

19.

A. Upper chambers of the heart are the right and left artia. (p. 209)

20.

A. There are four chambers in the human heart, which is located slightly left of the midline in the thoracic cavity. The upper chambers (atria) are separated by the interatrial septum, and the interventricular septum divides the two ventricles or lower chambers of the heart. (p. 209)

21.

C. The liquid portion of anticoagulated, or unclotted blood, is called plasma. It contains fibrinogen among other substances. (pp. 222–223)

22.

A. Serum does not contain anticoagulant. It is the fluid portion of a blood specimen that results when cellular components form a fibrin clot. Serum can be easily removed after centrifugation of the blood specimen. (p. 223)

23.

B. The cells sink to the bottom of the test tube after centrifugation because they are heavier than the liquid portion of the specimen. (p. 223)

24.

D. A thrombus is a blood clot. (p. 216)

25.

B. Arteriosclerosis, also called hardening of the arteries, is a condition whereby the artery becomes thickened and rough due to cholesterol buildup. (p. 216)

26.

D. Heart rate is measured by taking the pulse rate. (p. 213)

27.

D. The most common blood type is O. (p. 225)

28.

B. Transfusion reactions can occur if the wrong blood is transfused into a patient. The cells of the donor may react with the antibodies of the patient, causing hemolysis, agglutination, and clogging of small blood vessels as well as damage to kidneys, liver, lungs, heart, or the brain. These reactions can lead to death in some cases. (p. 226)

29.

C. A differential count refers to the enumeration of specific types of WBCs. (p. 227)

30.

D. The carotid arteries supply blood to the head and neck regions. (p. 214)

31.

A. The brachial artery is the major artery in the antecubital area of the arm. (p. 214)

32.

A. The median cubital vein is the most commonly used vein for venipuncture because it is generally the largest, closest to the surface of the skin, and best-anchored vein. (p. 219)

33.

B. The term "buffy coat" refers to the layer of WBCs and platelets that form when plasma is centrifuged or if the cells are allowed to settle. It forms above the RBC layer and below the plasma. (p. 223)

34.

A. If a patient is on Coumadin or other anticoagulant therapy, the phlebotomist should be on the alert that the patient might bleed more than usual due to slowed blood clotting. (p. 227)

35.

A. Hemostasis is a complex series of processes in which platelets, plasma, and coagulation factors interact to control bleeding while at the same time maintaining circulating blood in the liquid state. (pp. 233–234)

36.

D. The term "fibrinolysis" refers to the final phase of hemostasis, whereby repair and regeneration of the injured vessel take place, and the blood clot slowly begins to dissolve as other cells carry out further repair. (p. 234)

37.

B. Laboratory tests for blood typing and cross-matching for donor blood are performed in the immunohematology laboratory. (p. 228)

38.

D. The reference range for platelets is 250,000–500,000/mm^3. (p. 214)

39.

D. Hemophilia is a disease that can cause excessive bleeding due to abnormalities or suppressed clotting factors. (pp. 236–237)

40.

A. The longest vein in the body is the greater saphenous. It extends the length of the leg. (p. 215)

41.

B. Bone marrow is aspirated from the iliac crest of the hip. A physician performs the aspiration. These specimens are studied microscopically for the detection of abnormal numbers and characteristics of blood cells. (p. 228)

42.

A. Coagulation tests are performed for presurgical workups, among other reasons. (p. 237)

43.

A. Platelet functions as well as each coagulation factor can be measured from anticoagulated blood specimens in the coagulation section of the clinical hematology laboratory. (pp. 228–229)

44.

B. Since hemoglobin is contained within the erythrocytes or RBCs, they must be lysed to release the hemoglobin for assessment. (p. 224)

For Questions 45–50, refer to Figure 7.1.

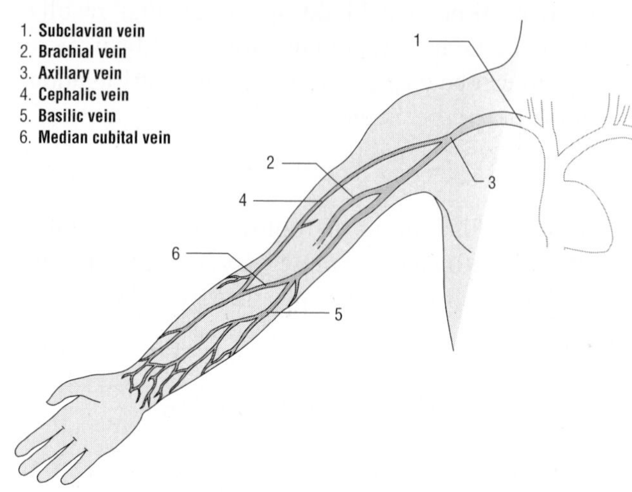

45.

A. "1" most closely resembles the subclavian vein. (p. 219)

46.

D. "2" most closely resembles the brachial vein. (p. 219)

47.

B. "3" most closely resembles the axillary vein. (p. 219)

48.

C. "4" most closely resembles the cephalic vein. (p. 219)

49.

D. "5" most closely resembles the basilic vein. (p. 219)

50.

A. "6" most closely resembles the median cubital vein. (p. 219)

CHAPTER

8 Blood Collection Equipment

chapter objectives

Upon completion of Chapter 8, the learner is responsible for the following:

1. Describe the latest phlebotomy safety supplies and equipment, and evaluate their effectiveness in blood collection.
2. List the various types of anticoagulants and additives used in blood collection, their mechanisms of action on collected blood, examples of tests performed on these tubes, and the vacuum-collection-tube color codes for these anticoagulants and additives.
3. Identify the various supplies that should be carried on a specimen collection tray when collecting blood by venipuncture or skin puncture.
4. Identify the types of safety equipment needed to collect blood by venipuncture and skin puncture.

DIRECTIONS Each of the questions or incomplete statements below is followed by four suggested answers or completions. Select one answer that is best in each case.

1. The device shown in Figure 8.1 can be used to collect specimens for:
   A. blood cultures
   B. hematocrit
   C. glucose tolerance test (GTT)
   D. venous glucose testing

2. John, a phlebotomist who collects only capillary blood from patients in the newborn and pediatric units, would probably have all of the following equipment on his blood collection tray except:
   A. BD blood transfer device
   B. sterile gauze pads

FIGURE 8.1

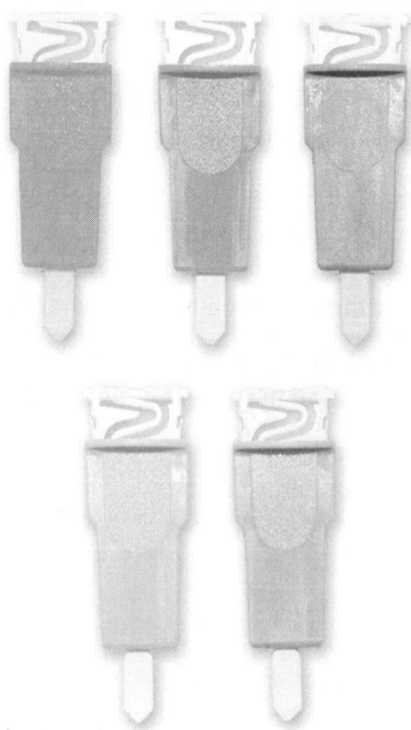

   C. BD Unopettes
   D. biohazardous waste container for sharps

3. Blood for lead levels needs to be collected in a:
   A. light-blue-topped tube
   B. purple-topped tube
   C. tan-topped tube
   D. green-topped tube

4. Which of the following is the best for the sterile blood collection of trace elements, toxicology, and nutritional studies?
   A. gold-topped tube
   B. royal-blue-topped tube
   C. purple-topped tube
   D. yellow-topped tube

5. The device shown in Figure 8.2 is the:
   A. BD Eclipse blood collection needle
   B. Sarstedt S-Monovette venous blood collection system

FIGURE 8.2 Courtesy and Copyright Becton, Dickinson and Company.

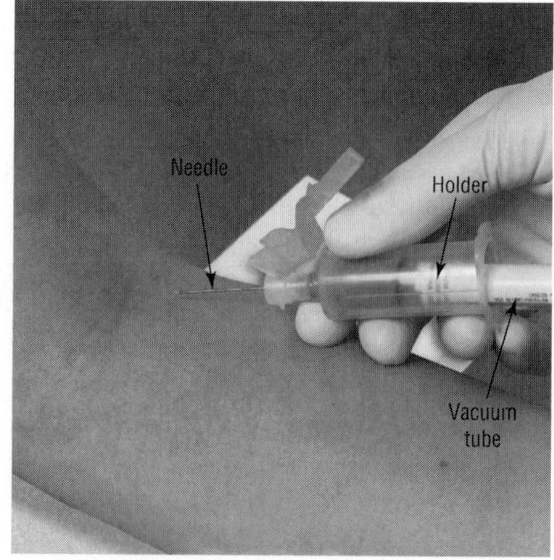

C. Vanishpoint blood collection tube holder

D. Venipuncture Needle-Pro needle protection device

6. The darker tubes shown in Figure 8.3 are needed in the collection of blood to test for:

A. glucose

B. enzymes

C. bilirubin

D. hematocrit

7. The glycolytic inhibitor is found in the:

A. green-topped tube

B. purple-topped tube

C. gray-topped tube

D. light-blue-topped tube

8. The blood collection set shown in Figure 8.4 is frequently used with the needle gauge size of:

A. 23

B. 19

C. 18

D. 17

9. For newborns, the penetration depth of lancets for blood collection must be less than:

A. 3.0 mm

B. 2.8 mm

C. 2.4 mm

D. 2.0 mm

FIGURE 8.3 Courtesy of Terumo Medical Corp., Somerset, NJ.

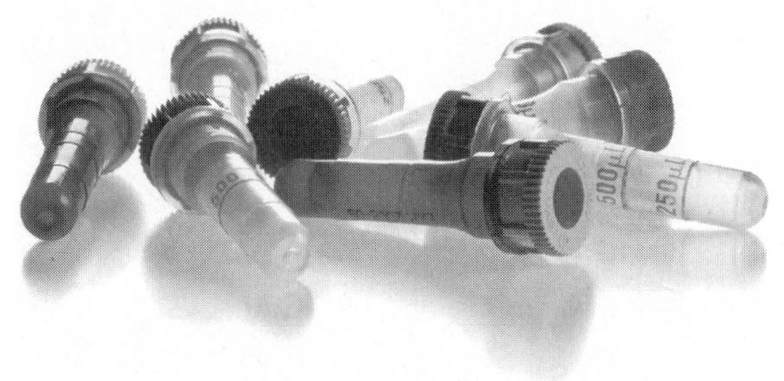

FIGURE 8.4 Courtesy of Becton, Dickinson and Company.

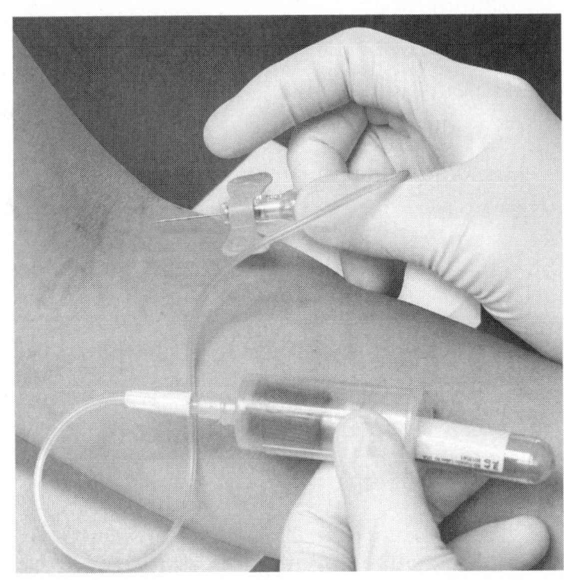

10. Which of the following anticoagulants is found in a lavender-topped blood collection vacuum tube?

A. ammonium heparin

B. sodium heparin

C. EDTA

D. sodium oxalate

11. Which of the following additives prevents the coagulation of blood by removing calcium through the formation of insoluble calcium salts?

A. ammonium oxalate, EDTA, sodium heparin

B. EDTA, lithium heparin, sodium citrate

C. sodium fluoride, lithium heparin, EDTA

D. EDTA, sodium citrate, potassium oxalate

12. Which of the following anticoagulants is found in a green-topped blood collection vacuum tube?
    A. EDTA
    B. potassium oxalate
    C. sodium citrate
    D. sodium heparin

13. Which of the following contains an antiglycolytic agent?
    A. light-blue-topped tube
    B. purple-topped tube
    C. gray-topped tube
    D. green-topped tube

14. A blood cell count requires whole blood collected in a:
    A. green-topped tube
    B. lavender-topped tube
    C. gray-topped tube
    D. light-blue-topped tube

15. The Monoject Monoletter is a:
    A. safety device for collecting arterial blood gas (ABG) specimens
    B. safety device for collecting specimens by venipuncture
    C. safe method to dispose of sharps
    D. safety device for collecting capillary blood

16. Specimens for which of the following tests must be collected in light-blue-topped blood collection tubes?
    A. APTT
    B. RPR test
    C. VDRL
    D. selenium

17. Criteria used to describe vacuum collection tube size are:
    A. external tube diameter, maximum amount of specimen to be collected, and external tube length
    B. external tube diameter, minimum amount of specimen that can be collected, and external tube length
    C. internal tube diameter, maximum amount of specimen to be collected, and external tube length
    D. internal tube diameter, minimum amount of specimen that can be collected, and internal tube length

18. Figure 8.5 shows which of the following?
    A. S-Monovette® venous blood collection system
    B. Vanishpoint blood collection tube holder

FIGURE 8.5 Courtesy of Sarstedt, Inc., Newton, NC.

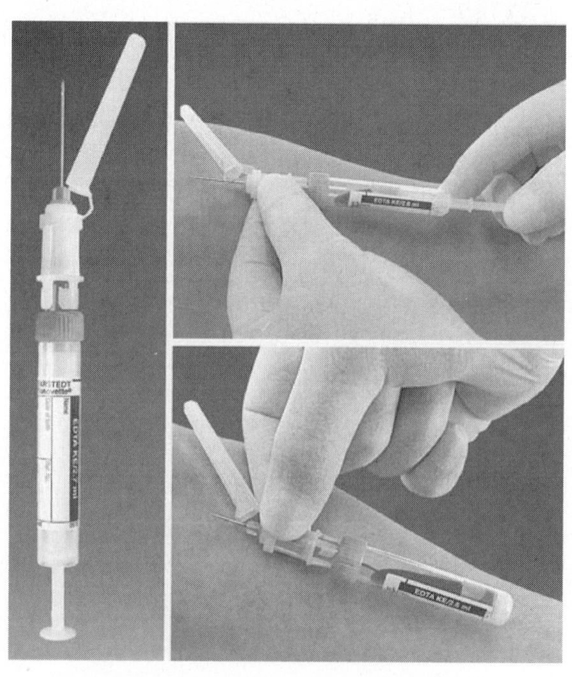

C. BD Eclipse blood collection needle Set
D. Venipuncture Needle-Pro needle protection device

19. Which of the following is a commonly used intravenous device that is sometimes used in the collection of blood from patients who are difficult to collect blood by conventional methods?
    A. Microvette® capillary blood collection system
    B. BD Unopette
    C. Surshield safety winged blood collection set
    D. BD Microtainer

20. What anticoagulant is preferred for the collection of whole blood in order to collect blood for STAT situations in clinical chemistry?
    A. heparin
    B. sodium citrate
    C. EDTA
    D. sodium oxalate

21. The blood collection device shown in Figure 8.6 can be used for:
    A. microcollection of blood for sed rate
    B. ABO grouping and typing blood collection
    C. microcollection and dilution of blood samples for the WBC count
    D. microcollection of blood for culture and sensitivity testing

22. Which of the following best describes Figure 8.7?
    A. safety device for collecting ABG specimens
    B. safe method to transfer capillary blood
    C. safety blood transfer device for venous specimens
    D. safety prefilled device used as a transfer and dilution unit

FIGURE 8.6 Courtesy of Becton, Dickinson and Company.

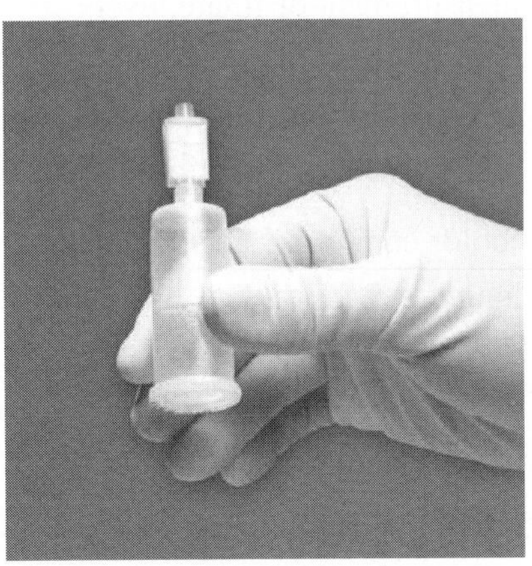

FIGURE 8.7 Courtesy of Becton, Dickinson and Company.

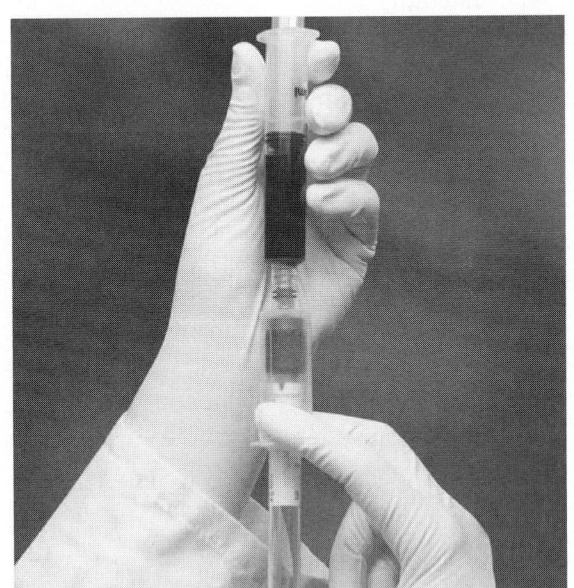

23. A prefilled device used as a collection and dilution unit is the:
    A. BD Unopette
    B. Vacuette tube
    C. heparinized microcollection tube
    D. Safe-T-Fill capillary blood collection device

24. The anticoagulant lithium heparin is most appropriate for blood collection to perform:
    A. measurement of folate levels
    B. measurement of potassium levels
    C. measurement of lithium levels
    D. blood smear preparations

25. The color coding for needles indicates the:
    A. length
    B. manufacturer
    C. gauge size
    D. anticoagulant

26. Which of the following blood analytes is sensitive to light?
    A. lead
    B. glucose
    C. calcium
    D. bilirubin

27. Which of the following anticoagulants is used frequently in coagulation blood studies?
    A. citrate–phosphate–dextrose (CPD)
    B. potassium oxalate
    C. acid–citrate–dextrose (ACD)
    D. sodium citrate

28. Figure 8.8 shows the:
    A. Sarstedt S-Monovette venous blood collection system
    B. Vanishpoint blood collection tube holder
    C. Venipuncture Needle-Pro needle protection device
    D. Vacuette Quickshield safety tube holder

29. When blood is collected from a patient, the serum should be separated from the blood cells as quickly as possible to avoid:
    A. hemoconcentration
    B. hemolysis
    C. glycolysis
    D. hemostasis

FIGURE 8.8 Courtesy of Retractable Technologies, Little Elm, TX.

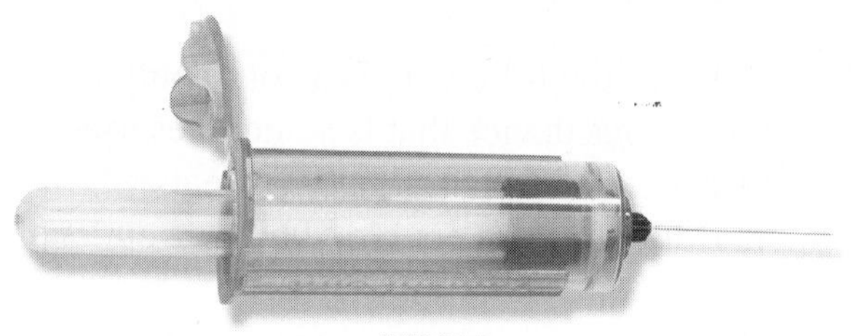

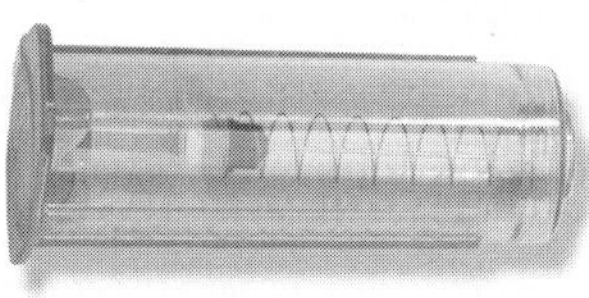

30. The yellow-topped vacuum collection tube has which of the following additives?
    A. EDTA
    B. lithium heparin
    C. trisodium citrate
    D. sodium polyanetholesulfonate (SPS)

31. Which of the following tests usually requires blood collected in a tan-topped blood collection vacuum tube?
    A. cortisol level
    B. CBC level
    C. lactate dehydrogenase level
    D. lead level

32. The evacuated tube system requires:
    A. a special safety plastic adapter, a safety syringe, and an evacuated sample tube
    B. an evacuated sample tube, a safety plastic adapter, and a double-pointed needle
    C. a double-pointed needle, a plastic safety holder, and a winged infusion set
    D. a special safety plastic adapter, an anticoagulant, and a double-pointed needle

33. To avoid microclotting in the blood collection tube, it is extremely important that the blood collected in a lavender-topped tube be gently inverted a minimum of:
    A. 0 times
    B. 5 times
    C. 8 times
    D. 12 times

34. The vial shown in Figure 8.9 is used in the collection of:
    A. microscopy specimens
    B. microbiology specimens
    C. clinical immunology specimens
    D. clinical chemistry specimens

FIGURE 8.9 Courtesy of Becton, Dickinson and Company.

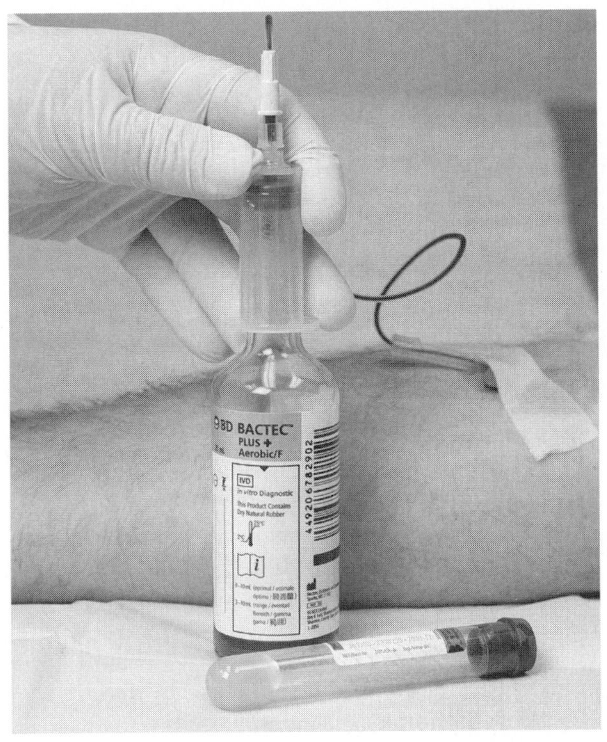

35. Measurement of blood copper, a trace element, requires blood collection in a:
    A. light-blue-topped tube
    B. green-topped tube
    C. royal-blue-topped tube
    D. purple-topped tube

36. Which of the following containers is frequently used for the micromeasurement of packed red cell volume?
    A. BD Unopette
    B. microhematocrit tube
    C. BD Microtainer
    D. S-Monovette blood collection system

37. The bleeding time assay is used to:
    A. access the RBC formation in the blood vessels
    B. access the contributions of platelet function and blood vessel integrity to blood clotting
    C. test the contributions of WBC and platelet formation in blood clotting activity
    D. measure the capability of platelets and Factor V to cause blood clotting

38. Which of the listed needle gauges has the smallest diameter?
    A. 19
    B. 20
    C. 21
    D. 23

39. Which of the following anticoagulants allows preparation of blood films with minimal distortion of WBCs?
    A. lithium heparin
    B. sodium citrate
    C. EDTA
    D. sodium heparin

40. Which of the following devices was developed specifically for the bleeding time assay?
    A. Tenderlett
    B. Autolet Lite Clinisafe
    C. Surgicutt
    D. Unopette

41. Which of the following is an anticoagulant used in blood donations?
    A. sodium citrate
    B. ACD
    C. EDTA
    D. lithium iodoacetate

42. If the phlebotomist collects only venipuncture specimens, which of the following items would *not* be needed on his or her specimen collection tray?
    A. disposable gloves
    B. tourniquet
    C. alcohol, iodine, and chlorhexidine swabs
    D. Tenderletts

43. Cytogenetic analysis requires whole blood collected in a:
    A. green-topped tube
    B. red-topped tube
    C. gray-topped tube
    D. light-blue-topped tube

44. The BD Unopette is:
    A. an amber-colored microcollection container to collect blood for bilirubin measurement
    B. a microdilution system
    C. used in the GTT microcollection
    D. a Mylar-wrapped glass capillary tube containing lithium heparin

45. The red and black speckled-topped blood collection tube should be gently inverted five times so that blood clotting occurs in:
    A. 5 minutes
    B. 15 minutes
    C. 30 minutes
    D. 45 minutes

46. The phlebotomist traveled to the home of 85-year-old Mrs. Ruth Harrison to collect blood for the PT, APTT, and potassium levels. Even though the blood collection was performed on Mrs. Harrison's fragile veins using a winged infusion set, the light-blue-topped tube was underfilled. However, the required amount of blood was collected in the green-topped tube. Which of the following will most likely occur?
    A. The potassium value will be falsely elevated.
    B. The PT and PTT results will be falsely prolonged.
    C. The potassium value will be falsely decreased.
    D. The PT and PTT results will not be affected.

47. The device shown in Figure 8.10 is:
    A. used in the collection of blood for the bleeding time procedure
    B. an instrument that provides a noninvasive procedure to visualize veins
    C. an instrument used in conjunction with disposable sterile lancets for the collection of microhematocrits
    D. occasionally used instead of a tourniquet in blood collection

48. A minimal volume of blood should be collected from a person to avoid the risk of iatrogenic:
    A. leukemia
    B. lymphoma

FIGURE 8.10 Courtesy of Venoscope, LLC, Lafayette, Louisiana.

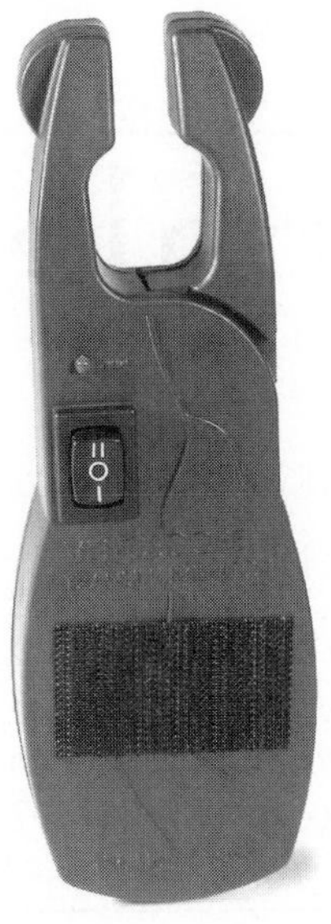

C. anemia
D. polycythemia

49. Which of the following anticoagulants is found in a royal-blue-topped blood collection tube?
    A. lithium heparin
    B. no anticoagulant
    C. sodium citrate
    D. ammonium heparin

50. Lithium heparin is a suitable anticoagulant for which of the following studies?
    A. erythrocyte sedimentation rate
    B. zinc level
    C. glucose level
    D. lithium level

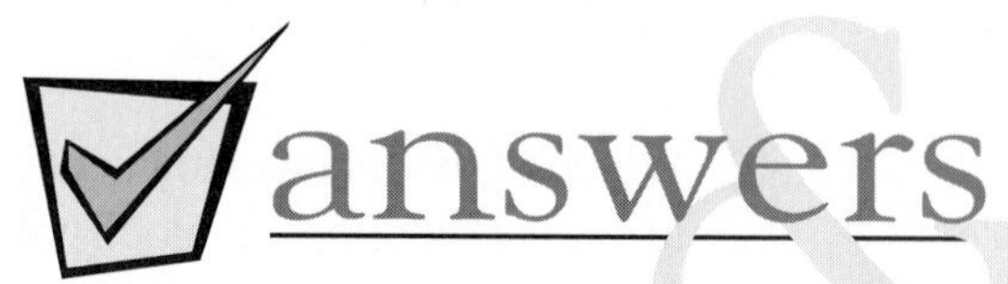

answers & rationales

1.

B. The device shown in Figure 8.1 can be used to collect specimens for hematocrit testing. (p. 271)

2.

A. John, a phlebotomist who collects only capillary blood from patients in the newborn and pediatric units, would probably have BD Unopettes, sterile gauze pads, and a biohazardous waste container but not the BD blood transfer device. (p. 258)

3.

C. The tan-topped tube has been designed for the blood collection of lead determinations. (p. 257)

4.

B. The royal-blue-topped tube has been designed to collect blood specimens for the determination of trace elements, toxicology, and/or nutritional studies. (p. 257)

5.

A. Figure 8.2 shows the BD Eclipse blood collection needle. (p. 259)

6.

C. The darker tubes shown in Figure 8.3 are needed in the collection of blood to test for bilirubin. (p. 271)

7.

C. The gray-topped tube contains a glycolytic inhibitor used in glucose testing. (p. 257)

8.

A. The blood collection set shown in Figure 8.4 is frequently used with the needle gauge size of 23. (pp. 262–263)

9.

D. For newborns, lancets with tips less than 2.0 mm are required to avoid penetrating bone. (p. 269)

10.

C. The anticoagulant EDTA is found in a lavender-topped blood collection vacuum tube. (p. 256)

11.

D. Coagulation of blood can be prevented by the addition of oxalates, citrates, and/or EDTA by their ability to remove calcium through the formation of insoluble calcium salts. (p. 253)

12.

D. The anticoagulant sodium heparin is found in a green-topped blood collection vacuum tube. (p. 255)

13.

C. The gray-topped tube contains sodium fluoride or lithium iodoacetate, which are antiglycolytic agents. (p. 257)

14.

B. A blood cell count, including WBC count, RBC count, hemoglobin (Hgb), hematocrit (Hct), mean corpuscular volume (MCV), mean corpuscular hemoglobin (MCH), and mean corpuscular hemoglobin concentration (MCHC), requires whole blood collected in a lavender-topped blood collection tube. (p. 256)

15.

D. The Monoject Monoletter is a safety device for skin puncture. (p. 270)

16.

A. The APTT requires blood collection in the light-blue-topped tubes containing citrate. (p. 254)

17.

A. The external tube diameter and length and the maximum amount of specimen that can be collected into the vacuum tube are the criteria that are used to describe vacuum collection tube size. (p. 251)

18.

A. Figure 8.5 shows the Sarstedt S-Monovette venous blood collection system. (p. 261)

19.

C. The butterfly needle, also referred to as a winged infusion set, is the most commonly used intravenous device. (p. 264)

20.

A. Heparinized whole blood has become the specimen of choice for the clinical chemistry instruments used in STAT situations. (p. 255)

21.

C. The blood collection device shown in Figure 8.6 can be used for microcollection and dilution of blood samples for the WBC count. (pp. 272–273)

22.

C. Figure 8.7 shows a safety blood transfer device for venous specimens. (p. 258)

23.

A. The BD Unopette is a blood collection device that is prefilled with specific amounts of diluents or reagents. (pp. 233–234)

24.

B. For potassium measurements, heparinized plasma or whole blood, rather than serum, is preferred. (pp. 255–256)

25.

C. The gauge size of the needle is identified by the color code on the sealed shield. (p. 259)

26.

D. Bilirubin breaks down chemically when exposed to light, and thus, the blood must be protected from light when bilirubin is to be measured. (p. 271)

27.

D. Sodium citrate, the anticoagulant in light-blue-topped blood collection tubes, is frequently used in coagulation blood studies. (p. 254)

28.

B. Figure 8.8 shows the Vanishpoint blood collection tube holder. (p. 260)

29.

C. Glycolysis is the breakdown of glucose, which can lead to erroneously low blood glucose results if the RBCs are not separated from the serum. (p. 257)

30.

D. SPS is used in the collection of blood culture specimens. (p. 253)

31.

D. Lead levels in blood are very minute and require a blood collection tube without any detectable lead such as the tan-topped tube. (p. 257)

32.

B. The evacuated tube system requires three components: an evacuated sample tube, a special safety plastic adapter, and a double-pointed needle. (pp. 250–251)

33.

C. The lavender-topped tube must be gently inverted at least eight times after blood collection to prevent clotting. (p. 256)

34.

D. The BD BACTEC culture vials shown in Figure 8.9 are used for microbiology blood collections. (p. 254)

35.

C. The royal-blue-topped tube is designed for the collection of trace elements such as copper. (p. 257)

36.

B. The microhematocrit tube contains heparin and is used for the collection of specimens to measure packed RBC volume. (p. 270)

37.

B. The bleeding time assay is used to access the contributions of platelet function and blood vessel integrity to blood clotting. (p. 266)

38.

D. The smaller the gauge number, the larger the diameter of the needle. (p. 259)

39.

C. EDTA is used to collect blood for blood smears, since it creates minimal distortion of WBCs. (p. 253)

40.

C. Surgicutt is a sterile, standardized, disposable instrument that is used for bleeding time assay. (p. 266)

41.

B. ACD is one of the anticoagulants that is used extensively in blood donations. (p. 253)

42.

D. Tenderletts are safe, single-use, automatically retracting, disposable devices used for microcollection by skin puncture. (p. 270)

43.

A. Cytogenetic analysis usually requires whole blood collected in a green-topped (Na heparin) blood collection tube. (p. 256)

44.

B. The BD Unopette is a microdilution system. (pp. 272–273)

45.

C. The red and black speckled-topped blood collection tube should be gently inverted five times so that blood clotting occurs in 30 minutes. (p. 254)

46.

B. If a light-blue-topped tube is underfilled, coagulation results will be erroneously prolonged. (p. 254)

47.

B. The device shown in Figure 8.10 is an instrument that provides a noninvasive procedure to visualize veins. (p. 266)

48.

C. A minimal volume of blood should be collected from a person to avoid the risk of iatrogenic anemia. (p. 269)

49.

B. Royal-blue-topped tubes generally contain EDTA or no anticoagulant. (p. 252)

50.

C. Lithium heparin is found in green-topped tubes and is suitable for blood glucose measurements. (pp. 255–256)

CHAPTER

9 Preanalytical Complications Causing Medical Errors in Blood Collection

chapter objectives

Upon completion of Chapter 9, the learner is responsible for the following:

1. Describe preanalytical complications related to phlebotomy procedures and impacting patient safety.
2. Explain how to prevent and/or handle complications in blood collection.
3. List at least five factors about a patient's physical disposition (i.e., make-up) that can affect blood collection.
4. List examples of substances that can interfere in clinical analysis of blood constituents and describe methods used to prevent these interferences.
5. Describe how allergies, a mastectomy, edema, and thrombosis can affect blood collection.
6. List preanalytical complications that can arise with test requests and identification.
7. Describe complications associated with tourniquet pressure and fist pumping.

8. Identify how the preanalytical factors of syncope, petechiae, neurological complications, hemoconcentration, hemolysis, and intravenous therapy affect blood collection.
9. Describe methods used to prevent these interferences.

DIRECTIONS Each of the questions or incomplete statements below is followed by four suggested answers or completions. Select one answer that is best in each case.

1. A basal state exists:
   A. after the evening meal
   B. in the early morning, 12 hours after the last ingestion of food
   C. in the afternoon, 3 hours after ingestion of lunch
   D. before lunch
2. Which of the following should stop the health care worker from collecting blood from a patient's arm vein?
   A. high blood pressure
   B. cardiac bypass surgery
   C. stroke that occurred the previous morning
   D. mastectomy
3. If a blood specimen appears lipemic, it indicates that:
   A. the phlebotomist had performed excessive probing with the needle in the patient's arm
   B. RBCs have ruptured in the blood specimen
   C. triglycerides and/or cholesterol levels are elevated in the blood specimen
   D. the patient is in a basal state
4. Which of the following conditions is a falsely increased laboratory result for a blood analyte?
   A. Results are interpreted as normal, but the blood analyte is truly in an elevated range.
   B. Results are caused by a medication competing with the blood analyte for a chromogenic reagent, thus falsely decreasing the resultant color of the reaction.
   C. Results are interpreted as elevated or normal, but the blood analyte is truly in a normal or decreased range, respectively.
   D. The laboratory results are insignificant.
5. Which of the following has been shown to erroneously affect laboratory test results, leading to falsely elevated or decreased results?
   A. violent crying
   B. smiling
   C. syncope
   D. sneezing
6. If the phlebotomist is preparing to collect specimens for routine hematology, coagulation, and chemistry tests, and notices that the patient is taking aspirin, why should the phlebotomist be concerned?
   A. The patient may bleed excessively.
   B. The blood urea nitrogen (BUN) will be erroneous.
   C. The creatinine result will be altered.
   D. There is no cause for concern.
7. If a patient is overweight and the phlebotomist cannot access the vein when the needle is first inserted, what should the phlebotomist do?

A. Probe around until the vein is found.
B. Repalpate and adjust/move the needle slightly.
C. Push the needle all the way in because the vein is probably under layers of fat.
D. Give up the procedure and allow someone else to do it.

8. What is the effect on a patient if a phlebotomist punctures a nerve with the phlebotomy needle?
   A. It should not have an effect on the patient.
   B. It may tingle slightly but it should not interfere with the rest of the procedure.
   C. The specimen may be contaminated with interstitial fluid.
   D. The patient will feel a sharp radiating pain and the procedure should be discontinued.

9. When the phlebotomist collected blood from the patient, the patient was in a supine position. This means the patient was:
   A. lying down with his or her legs elevated
   B. sitting in a chair
   C. lying on his or her back
   D. standing near a counter

10. If a patient becomes extremely anxious and stressed during the blood collection procedure and begins to hyperventilate, which of the following laboratory results will be altered because of this stress?
    A. triglyceride level
    B. RBC count
    C. protein level
    D. blood pH level

11. What does Figure 9.1 depict?
    A. a hematoma appearing close to the antecubital fossa area
    B. a woman's arm showing lymphostasis
    C. petechiae close to the antecubital area
    D. a woman's arm showing hemoconcentration

FIGURE 9.1 Johnson & Johnson Medical Division, Inc, 1997 Used with permission of the copyright owner.

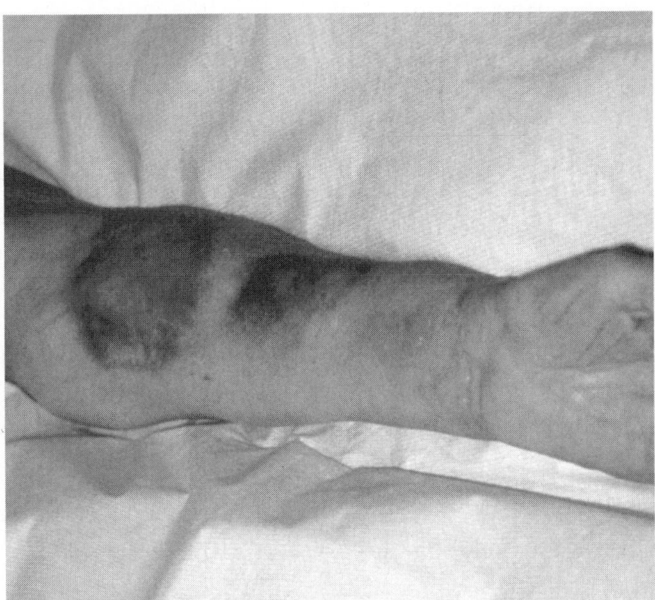

12. Effects of exercise have shown on blood laboratory tests an increase in:
    A. sodium
    B. total protein
    C. chloride
    D. carbon dioxide

13. What does the term "edema" mean?
    A. obesity
    B. infection of the skin
    C. buildup of fluid
    D. renal failure

14. Which of the following blood collection tubes is the most appropriate for use in transfusion medicine for cross-matching of blood?
    A. red-topped tube
    B. pink-topped tube
    C. red/grey-topped tube
    D. lavender-topped tube

15. As you met in the outpatient blood collection area with the outpatient Ms. Able, she mentioned that she had just smoked a cigarette and wanted to know if that would affect her blood test results. Which of the following blood analytes would you tell her that it would most likely lead to a falsely increased result?
    A. hemoglobin
    B. cholesterol
    C. RBCs
    D. bilirubin

16. During a venipuncture procedure, when the area around a venipuncture site starts to swell, this occurrence usually leads to:
    A. atherosclerosis
    B. lymphostasis
    C. hematoma formation
    D. petechiae formation

17. Solid mass(es) derived from blood constituents that occlude a blood vessel is/are:
    A. lymphostasis
    B. angiography
    C. thrombi
    D. petechiae

18. How long after a venipuncture procedure should pressure be applied to the puncture site?
    A. 30 seconds
    B. 60 seconds
    C. 90 seconds
    D. until the bleeding has stopped

19. If a patient that is having blood collected by you as the phlebotomist informs you that he just arrived home in the U.S. from China last night, what blood analyte values would most likely be affected?
    A. cortisol
    B. bilirubin
    C. chloride
    D. creatine kinase

20. If the phlebotomist is preparing to collect specimens for routine hematology, coagulation, and chemistry tests, and notices that the patient is on IV heparin therapy, why should the phlebotomist be concerned?
    A. The patient may bleed excessively.
    B. The BUN will be erroneous.
    C. The H and H will be altered.
    D. There is no cause for concern.

21. Which of the following occurs as a result of repeated punctures, inflammation, and disease of the interstitial compartments?
    A. hematoma
    B. hemoconcentration
    C. sclerosed veins
    D. syncope

22. Upon entering Mrs. Goethl's hospital room, the phlebotomist noticed that Mrs. Goethl was taking three aspirin tablets. The patient commented that she was taking a second dose of aspirin because the first dose she took last night did not help her headache. What blood test will most likely be affected by the aspirin intake?
    A. triglycerides
    B. glucose
    C. RBC count
    D. coagulation testing

23. If the tourniquet is incorrectly applied for longer than 3 minutes, which of the following blood analytes will most likely be falsely elevated?
    A. uric acid
    B. BUN
    C. potassium
    D. bilirubin

24. What does the term "preanalytical" refer to in phlebotomy practice?
    A. equipment malfunction prior to analytical testing
    B. when a test result is reported prior to verification of quality control parameters
    C. an episode of syncope
    D. variables that affect the specimen prior to laboratory analysis

25. Which of the following is the primary cause of vein collapse during venipuncture?
    A. Blood is withdrawn too quickly or forcefully.
    B. The tourniquet is not tight enough.
    C. The tourniquet is too tight.
    D. The tube has no vacuum in it.

26. Which of the following analytes is significantly increased in the blood with changes in position?
    A. testosterone
    B. glucose
    C. cortisol
    D. iron

27. Which of the following blood analytes is affected by diurnal rhythm?
    A. ACTH
    B. CK
    C. cholesterol
    D. creatinine

28. What effects do prolonged fasting or severe diets have on patients?
    A. No effects occur to the blood analytes.
    B. Only glucose tolerance levels are affected.
    C. Only WBC and RBC counts are affected.
    D. Electrolyte disturbances and cardiac dysrhythmias may result.

29. In most cases, when should blood be collected to determine blood levels of medications?
    A. at 7:00 AM
    B. at noon
    C. one hour after the medication is administered
    D. just prior to the next dose of the medication

30. Which of the following blood analytes increases with age?
    A. growth hormone
    B. estrogen
    C. cholesterol and triglycerides
    D. bilirubin

31. Another term for fainting is:
    A. syncope
    B. lymphostasis
    C. transient blood
    D. thrombus

32. What does the term "falsely decreased" laboratory result refer to?
    A. a laboratory result that is interpreted as subnormal even though the blood analyte is truly in an elevated or a normal range
    B. a laboratory result that is erroneously interpreted as normal
    C. a laboratory result caused by increasing the color produced in the laboratory test
    D. a laboratory result that does not have a significant impact on the patient's outcome

33. What is the ideal time for specimens to be collected?
    A. at noon if ingestion of food occurred at 8:00 AM
    B. 5 hours after the last ingestion of food
    C. 12 hours after the last ingestion of food
    D. 15 hours after the last ingestion of food

34. How many adults in the United States are overweight?
    A. less than 10%
    B. 20%
    C. more than 50%
    D. more than 90%

35. What does the term "occluded" mean in relation to veins?
    A. having larger diameter than normal
    B. inflamed due to an infection
    C. obstructed
    D. smaller than normal

36. Which of the following would most likely *not* be an explanation for turbid serum?
    A. elevated triglyceride results
    B. elevated cholesterol results
    C. bacterial contamination
    D. elevated glucose results

37. If a patient is allergic to iodine and alcohol, what could be used to disinfect the puncture site?
    A. chlorox
    B. sanitizing cleanser
    C. chlorhexidine
    D. soap and distilled water

38. What effect does hyperventilation have on laboratory values?
    A. increased blood glucose
    B. acid-base imbalances
    C. increased serum iron
    D. increased cell counts

39. What happens if a patient abstains from drinking water for 12–24 hours?
    A. The patient will maintain a basal state.
    B. The specimen will be somewhat diluted.
    C. The patient may become dehydrated.
    D. The glucose level would be elevated.

40. When hemoglobin is released and serum becomes tinged with pink or red, this condition is referred to as:
    A. lymphocytosis
    B. hemoconcentration
    C. hemolysis
    D. hemophilia

41. If a patient asks to chew sugarless gum prior to a fasting glucose procedure, what should the phlebotomist say?
    A. The phlebotomist should say that it is okay to chew sugarless gum.
    B. The phlebotomist should advise the patient to stop chewing the gum 15 minutes before the blood is collected for the blood glucose collection.
    C. The phlebotomist should say that it is okay to have coffee or tea but not gum.
    D. The phlebotomist should explain that chewing gum may cause a transient fluctuation in the blood sugar level.

42. Emotional stress, such as anxiety or fear of blood collections, can lead to an increase in:
    A. blood glucose
    B. RBC count
    C. WBC count
    D. serum iron

43. If the phlebotomist is preparing to collect specimens for routine hematology, coagulation, and chemistry tests, and notices that the patient is on IV Warfarin, why should the phlebotomist be concerned?
    A. The patient may bleed excessively.
    B. The BUN will be erroneous.
    C. The H and H will be altered.
    D. There is no cause for concern.

44. What effect does excessive probing with a needle in the patient's arm have on a venipuncture specimen?
    A. No effect at all and the specimen should be acceptable.
    B. It can rupture erythrocytes and release tissue-clotting factors.
    C. Probing is often necessary and alters only the leukocyte count.
    D. No effect, but a physician should be notified of the circumstances.

45. If blood is to be collected for a timed blood glucose level determination, the patient must fast for:
    A. 14–16 hours
    B. 8–12 hours
    C. 6–8 hours
    D. 4–6 hours

46. What is the most common cause of iron-deficiency anemia in women?
    A. excessive blood loss due to phlebotomy
    B. hemorrhage
    C. renal failure
    D. menstrual blood loss

47. If a phlebotomist collects a venipuncture specimen from an arm site slightly above the patient's IV (in the same arm), what effect does it have on the specimen?
    A. It will have no effect.
    B. It will increase the cellular counts.
    C. It will increase ammonia levels.
    D. It will dilute the specimen with IV fluids.

48. The phlebotomist assigned to collect a blood specimen from Ms. Pontius noticed that her right arm was swollen. She had recently had a mastectomy. This abnormal accumulation of fluid, localized or diffused, in the intercellular spaces of the body is referred to as:
    A. edema
    B. atherosclerosis
    C. hemolysis
    D. hemoconcentration

49. A physiological abnormality that can cause hemolysis is:
    A. needle readjustment
    B. performing blood collection before the alcohol has dried at the collection site
    C. sickle cell disease
    D. shaking blood collection tubes vigorously after blood collection

50. Why is it important to collect blood when the patient is in a basal state?
    A. It is most comfortable for the patient at this time.
    B. Laboratory tests are most reliable if the patient is in a basal state.
    C. Blood is thickest at this time.
    D. It fits well into the pre-established work schedules of most hospitals.

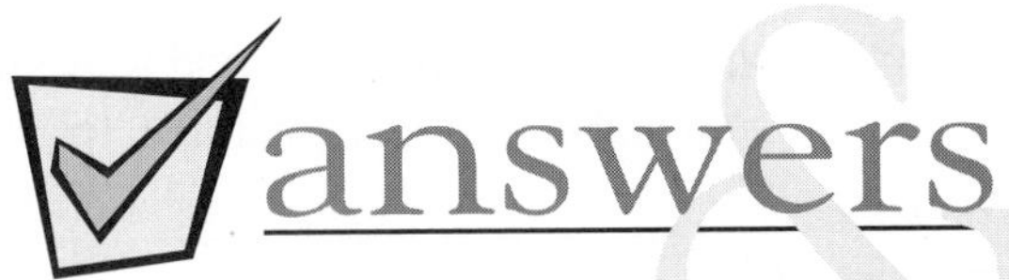

answers & rationales

1.

B. Basal state exists in the early morning, approximately 12 hours after the last ingestion of food. (p. 282)

2.

D. A woman or man who has had a mastectomy (removal of a breast) may also have lymphostasis due to lymph node removal adjacent to the breast. Without lymph flow on that particular side of the body, the patient is highly susceptible to infection, and some blood analytes may be altered. Therefore, venipuncture should *not* be performed on the same side as that of a mastectomy. (p. 287)

3.

C. If a blood specimen appears lipemic, it indicates that triglycerides and/or cholesterol levels are elevated in the blood specimen. (p. 283)

4.

C. Falsely increased laboratory test results for a blood analyte can be mistakenly interpreted as elevated or normal if the blood analyte is truly in a normal or decreased range, respectively. (p. 288)

5.

A. Violent crying can falsely alter laboratory test results dramatically. (p. 286)

6.

A. Aspirin may cause the patient to bleed excessively and will affect the coagulation test results. (p. 288)

7.

B. The needle should be adjusted slightly to try to find the vein. Usually these patients know where the best site is for venipuncture, so it is helpful to check with the patient prior to the procedure. (p. 284)

8.

D. If a phlebotomist punctures a patient's nerve with the phlebotomy needle, the patient is likely to feel a sharp, tingling, painful sensation that radiates down the nerve. The tourniquet should be released immediately, the needle removed, and pressure held over the blood collection site. An incident report about the occurrence should be completed and a supervisor notified. (p. 294)

9.

C. The term "supine" means that the patient was lying on his or her back. (p. 286)

10.

D. Anxiety that results in hyperventilation also causes acid-base imbalances, changing the blood pH level. (p. 286)

11.

A. This woman's arm shows a hematoma appearing close to the antecubital fossa area. A hematoma can occur when the needle has gone completely through a vein, the bevel opening is partially in the vein, or not enough pressure is applied to the site after puncture. (p. 293)

12.

B. The effects of exercise (e.g., running a marathon) have shown on blood laboratory tests increases in glucose, total protein, albumin, uric acid, calcium, phosphorus, BUN, creatinine, total and direct bilirubin, ALT, AST, and alkaline phosphatase. (p. 285)

13.

C. Edema refers to an abnormal accumulation of fluid in the intercellular spaces. It may be caused from a mastectomy, during heart or renal failure, or due to bacterial toxins or malnutrition. (p. 287)

14.

B. The pink-topped tube can be used in transfusion medicine (blood banking) for cross-matching of blood whereas the serum separator tubes, lavender-topped tubes, and red-topped tubes are not to be used for these procedures. (p. 296 and tube chart on the last page of the *Phlebotomy Handbook*, 8th ed.)

15.

B. The ingredients in cigarettes may affect several laboratory results. Through the action of nicotine from the tobacco, the blood concentrations of glucose, growth hormone, cholesterol, and triglycerides increase. (p. 288)

16.

C. When the area around the venipuncture site starts to swell, usually blood is leaking into the tissues and causing a hematoma. (p. 293)

17.

C. Thrombi are solid masses derived from blood constituents that reside in the blood vessels. (p. 284)

18.

D. Pressure should be applied to the venipuncture site until all of the bleeding has stopped. (p. 294)

19.

A. Communicating with the patient about recent long-distance travel is a controllable means for the health care worker to possibly avoid erroneous laboratory results. Since long-distance travel affects a person's circadian rhythm, it will affect cortisol results because cortisol and other hormones normally fluctuate with the daily circadian rhythm that is disrupted with travel over numerous time zones. (p. 286)

20.

A. Heparin therapy may cause the patient to bleed excessively and will affect the coagulation test results. (p. 288)

21.

C. Sclerosed, or hardened, veins are a result of inflammation and disease of the interstitial compartments after repeated venipunctures. (p. 284)

22.

D. Aspirin causes alterations in coagulation tests. (p. 288)

23.

C. The pressure of the tourniquet causes potassium to leak from the tissue cells into the blood, leading to its falsely elevated values if the tourniquet pressure is prolonged. (p. 290)

24.

D. In phlebotomy practice the term "preanalytical" refers to what happens to the specimen prior to laboratory analysis. Preanalytical variables can be controlled by the phlebotomist to minimize the risk of complications during or after the venipuncture procedure. (p. 282)

25.

A. The primary cause of vein collapse during venipuncture is that blood is withdrawn too quickly or forcefully. (p. 296)

26.

D. Changing from a lying position to a sitting or standing position causes body water to shift from intravascular to interstitial compartments (in tissues), and certain larger molecules such as iron cannot filter into the tissue. Thus they concentrate in the blood. (p. 286)

27.

A. Diurnal rhythms are body fluid fluctuations during the day that affect certain blood analytes such as ACTH. (p. 286)

28.

D. Prolonged fasting and/or severe diets to lose weight can cause health hazards including electrolyte disturbances, cardiac dysrhythmias, and even death. (p. 283)

29.

D. To determine levels of medications, blood should, in most cases, be collected just prior to the next dose. (p. 287)

30.

C. Blood cholesterol and triglyceride levels increase with age. (p. 286)

31.

A. Another term for fainting is syncope. (p. 292)

32.

A. Falsely decreased values of a blood analyte can be mistakenly interpreted as subnormal if the blood analyte is truly in an elevated or a normal range. (p. 288)

33.

C. The ideal time for specimens to be collected is in the early morning, approximately 12 hours after the last ingestion of food. (p. 282)

34.

C. More than half of adult patients in the United States are overweight. (p. 284)

35.

C. An occluded vein is obstructed and does not allow blood to flow through it. (p. 284)

36.

D. Turbid serum that appears cloudy or milky can be a result of bacterial contamination or high lipid (i.e., cholesterol, triglycerides) levels in the blood. Elevated glucose results should not cause the serum to appear turbid. (p. 283)

37.

C. If a patient is allergic to iodine and alcohol, chlorhexidine is an alternative to decontaminate the skin. It should be wiped off with sterile water after the application. (p. 284)

38.

B. Hyperventilation causes acid-base imbalances, increased lactate levels, and increased fatty acid levels. (p. 286)

39.

C. The patient may become dehydrated if he or she abstains from water for 12–24 hours. This can alter test results. It is important for the phlebotomist to explain the term "fasting" completely and ensure that the patient understands that they should abstain from food but not from water. (p. 283)

40.

C. Hemolysis is when the RBCs are lysed and release hemoglobin. (p. 295)

41.

D. The phlebotomist should explain that chewing gum may cause a transient fluctuation in the blood sugar level. Furthermore, the phlebotomist could offer the patient a glass of water and ask the patient to please wait until after the procedure to chew gum. (p. 283)

42.

C. Emotional stress, such as anxiety or fear of blood collection, can lead to an increase in the WBC count. (p. 285)

43.

A. Warfarin therapy may cause the patient to bleed excessively and will affect the coagulation test results. (p. 288)

44.

B. Excessive probing with a needle in the patient's arm can have a significant effect on a venipuncture specimen. It can cause rupturing of RBCs, increase the concentration of intracellular contents, and release some tissue-clotting factors. (p. 284)

45.

B. If blood is to be collected for a timed blood glucose level determination, the patient needs to fast for 8–12 hours. Prolonged fasting has been shown to falsely alter blood test results. (p. 283)

46.

D. Menstrual blood loss is the most common cause of iron-deficiency anemia in women. Thus, it is vitally important that phlebotomists not withdraw more blood than is absolutely necessary so as not to increase the negative effects of additional blood loss during venipuncture. (p. 287)

47.

D. If a phlebotomist collects a venipuncture specimen from an arm site slightly above the patient's IV, it will dilute the specimen with the IV fluid and result in erroneous results. (p. 294)

48.

A. An abnormal accumulation of fluid, localized or diffused, in the intercellular spaces of the body is referred to as edema. (p. 287)

49.

C. A physiological abnormality that can cause hemolysis is sickle cell disease. (p. 295)

50.

B. Basal state specimens are the most reliable ones. (p. 282)

CHAPTER

10 Venipuncture Procedures

chapter objectives

Upon completion of Chapter 10, the learner is responsible for the following:

1. Describe detailed steps in the patient identification process and what to do if information is missing.
2. Describe methods for hand hygiene.
3. Identify the most appropriate sites for venipuncture and situations when these sites might not be acceptable.
4. Identify alternative sites for the venipuncture procedure.
5. Describe the process and time limits for applying a tourniquet to a patient's arm.
6. Describe the decontamination process and the agents used to decontaminate skin for routine blood tests and blood cultures.
7. Describe the steps of a venipuncture procedure using the evacuated tube method, syringe method, and butterfly method according to the CLSI Approved Standard.
8. Describe the "order of draw" for collection tubes.

9. Explain the clinical reason for collecting "timed specimens" at the requested times.
10. Define the terms *fasting* and *STAT* when referring to blood tests.

DIRECTIONS Each of the questions or incomplete statements below is followed by four suggested answers or completions. Select one answer that is best in each case.

1. When describing hand-hygiene and gloving procedures, which of the statements is accurate prior to a venipuncture procedure?
   A. Hand hygiene is more important than gloving.
   B. Gloving is more important than hand hygiene.
   C. After cleansing hands thoroughly there is no need to wear gloves.
   D. Good hand hygiene does not eliminate the need to wear gloves.
2. Prior to performing a venipuncture, why should a clean pair of gloves be put on in the presence of the patient?
   A. It is a federal law for all health care workers.
   B. It is a reassuring, safety-conscious gesture for both the patient and the worker.
   C. It saves time and money.
   D. It eliminates the need for repeated hand-hygiene techniques.
3. What is the importance of hand-hygiene techniques?
   A. It significantly reduces the number of outbreaks of infections.
   B. It prevents HBV infection after a needlestick.
   C. It helps with vein selection.
   D. It eliminates the use of gloves.
4. What does MRSA signify?
   A. Multiple Reasons for Safety Advice
   B. Methicillin Resistant *Staphylococcus aureus*
   C. Measures of Radiation Alert
   D. Mumps and Rubella Serum Antibodies
5. Identification of an inpatient can *best* be accomplished by which of the following?
   A. using the patient's hospital identification bracelet and a verbal confirmation from the patient
   B. hospital room number and bed assignment
   C. confirmation from a patient's relative
   D. matching the patient's hospital identification bracelet, test request information, and a verbal confirmation
6. Information on an inpatient's identification armband always includes the:
   A. patient's name and identification number
   B. physician's name and laboratory tests usually ordered
   C. patient's bed assignment
   D. nearest relative and emergency phone number

7. If an inpatient is semiconscious, has severe burns, and does not have an identification bracelet, who would be the best person to ask to make the identification before a venipuncture?
   A. the patient's cousin who is visiting him or her
   B. another patient in the room
   C. the clerk who checked the patient in
   D. the nurse in charge of the patient

8. Which of the following item(s) of information is *not* a requirement for laboratory test requisitions (electronic or handwritten)?
   A. patient's full name, identification number, and date of birth
   B. dates and types of tests to be performed
   C. physician's name
   D. social security number and password

9. If a phlebotomist is assigned to collect a blood specimen from an outpatient named Susan Long, which of the following statements is the best way to ask for the patient's name?
   A. Good morning, Mrs. Long. Did you eat breakfast today?
   B. Are you Susan Long?
   C. Could you please confirm that your name is Susan Long?
   D. Could you please state your name and spell it for me?

10. Hand lotions can be used in phlebotomy for which of the following purposes?
    A. to finish the process of hand antisepsis
    B. to maximize antiseptic action
    C. to minimize the occurrence of dermatitis
    D. to provide lubrication prior to wearing gloves

11. What type of hand sanitizer is usually acceptable for decontamination of hands prior to a venipuncture procedure?
    A. saline-based
    B. alcohol-based
    C. rubs that are slightly acidic
    D. lotion-based

12. How much hand sanitizer is needed to decontaminate hands?
    A. 0.5 mL
    B. 1 mL
    C. 5 mL
    D. the amount that is recommended by the manufacturer

13. What should a phlebotomist do if his or her hands are visibly dirty with dust and dirt?
    A. Wash hands with soap and water.
    B. Use an alcohol-based hand rub and wipe it off with paper towels.
    C. Use antimicrobial wipes.
    D. Wear sterile gloves.

14. If a phlebotomist accidentally sticks himself or herself with a contaminated needle, what is the first thing he should do?
    A. Immediately wash the area with soap and water.
    B. Call a supervisor.
    C. Test the patient for HIV and HBV.
    D. Proceed with routine tasks and report it during the next break.

15. Which of the following is the most common site for venipuncture?
    A. median cubital vein
    B. ulnar vein
    C. basilic vein
    D. radial vein

16. Select one reason for not using arm veins for a venipuncture?
    A. The patient has IV lines or casts on both arms.
    B. The patient is a child and is temperamental.
    C. The patient is an older person and tends to fall asleep during the procedure.
    D. The patient is frail and in pain.

17. If arm veins cannot be used for a venipuncture, the preferred alternative veins lie in the:
    A. ankles or feet
    B. anterior surface of the hand or wrist
    C. dorsal side of the hand or wrist
    D. outermost edge of the hand

18. Which of the following does *not* need to be included on the label of the blood or body fluid specimen?
    A. patient's name and identification number
    B. the time that the specimen is collected
    C. the attending physician's name
    D. social security number and password

19. What happens if the tourniquet pressure is too tight or prolonged on the arm prior to the venipuncture?
    A. Laboratory test results may be affected due to hemoconcentration.
    B. Laboratory test results will not be affected.
    C. Only drug levels will be falsely decreased.
    D. Tourniquet pressure will cause excessive bleeding after the procedure.

20. Where should the tourniquet be placed on the patient during the venipuncture procedure?
    A. 1–2 inches above the venipuncture site
    B. 1–2 inches underneath the venipuncture site
    C. 3–4 inches above the venipuncture site
    D. 3–4 inches underneath the venipuncture site

21. Which of the following causes pooling of blood in veins?
    A. syringe method
    B. tourniquet
    C. capillary tube
    D. evacuated tube method

22. After a venipuncture site has been cleansed with alcohol, which of the following is the appropriate step?
    A. Blow on the site to speed the drying process.
    B. Using the gloved hand, fan the site to assist in drying.
    C. Allow the site to air-dry.
    D. Continue immediately with the venipuncture.

23. If a patient is allergic to alcohol, what is an acceptable alternate cleansing agent?
    A. saline
    B. chlorhexidine compounds
    C. 1:10 dilution of chlorox
    D. 30% isopropanol

24. During the venipuncture, what is the best angle for inserting the needle into the skin?
    A. 30 degrees or less
    B. 45–60 degrees
    C. 60–80 degrees
    D. 90 degrees

25. During a normal venipuncture procedure, after the needle is inserted and blood begins to flow, what should the phlebotomist do next?
    A. Release the tourniquet.
    B. Withdraw the needle.
    C. Release the adapter.
    D. Adjust the hub of the needle.

26. When the evacuated tube method is used for venipuncture, which one of the following is the correct order of collection for the following tubes (by their color of tube top): blood culture tubes, coagulation tube, and hematology tube?
    A. light blue, lavender, yellow blood culture tubes
    B. lavender, light blue, yellow blood culture tubes
    C. yellow blood culture tubes, light blue, lavender
    D. light blue, yellow blood culture tubes, lavender

27. When using a butterfly needle set to collect a specimen for a single coagulation test, which of the following is an essential step?
    A. Make a notation on the specimen label about the method of collection.
    B. Draw a discard tube first.
    C. Withdraw a dummy tube after the specimen is collected.
    D. Split the blood specimen into two tubes.

28. When describing phlebotomy procedures, the term "STAT" refers to:
    A. abstaining from food over a period of time
    B. using timed blood collections for specific specimens
    C. using the early morning specimens for laboratory testing
    D. immediate and urgent specimen collection

29. Overfilling a citrate tube with blood can cause which of the following effects?
    A. hemolysis
    B. hemoconcentration
    C. falsely shortened clotting times
    D. falsely elevated hemoglobin levels

30. Why is it important to get information about whether or not the patient has recently eaten?
    A. Laboratory tests can be affected by the ingestion of food and drink.
    B. Meals will likely make the patient vomit during the procedure.
    C. After eating, patients usually have enlarged veins.
    D. It is not that important to get this information.

31. How often should a health care worker perform hand-hygiene procedures when many patients' venipunctures need to be performed during a short period of time?
    A. after every two patients
    B. after every five patients
    C. at the beginning and end of a shift
    D. before and after each patient

32. If a patient is obese, what special equipment would be most helpful in the specimen collection process?
    A. specially sized collection tubes and ice packs
    B. a face mask and gown
    C. a large-sized blood pressure cuff and longer needle
    D. a large-sized wheelchair and warming blankets

33. The recommended way to locate a vein for a routine venipuncture is which of the following?
    A. slight elevation of the patient's arm
    B. palpating the entire antecubital area to feel the vein
    C. to see the vein close to the skin surface
    D. asking the doctor for a preferred site

34. Which of the following procedures reduces the potential for hazards when performing a venipuncture procedure using the syringe method?
    A. Collect the specimen from the wrist.
    B. Use a blood transfer device to expel blood into the tubes.
    C. Leave the tourniquet on for up to 2 minutes.
    D. Push the plunger quickly to rapidly get blood into the tubes.

35. Arteries differ from veins in which of the following ways?
    A. thicker vessel walls with a pulsating feel
    B. more visible to the eye
    C. smaller in diameter
    D. have warmer blood than the veins

36. If a patient has had a mastectomy on his or her right side, what venipuncture site should be considered first?
    A. the antecubital area of the right arm
    B. the antecubital area of the left arm
    C. the dorsal side of the right hand
    D. the dorsal side of the left hand

37. During a venipuncture procedure, the needle should always be inserted with the:
    A. bevel side down
    B. bevel side up
    C. bevel pointed away from the insertion site
    D. bevel perpendicular to the skin

38. If a phlebotomist cannot successfully perform a venipuncture at the first attempt, what should he or she do?
    A. Use a smaller needle next time.
    B. Switch to a syringe method.
    C. Check for a different site and if it feels palpable, try only one more time.
    D. Keep trying until he or she is successful.

39. The winged infusion set is useful and preferred for venipunctures in all but which one of the listed situations?
    A. young adult males
    B. small hand or wrist veins
    C. young children
    D. severely burned patients

40. After withdrawing a needle from a patient's arm, what step should be performed *immediately?*
    A. activating the safety device on the needle
    B. applying an adhesive bandage to the site
    C. labeling the specimen
    D. disposing of the needle

41. On occasion, specimens may be rejected for laboratory testing. Which of the following would be a likely cause for specimen rejection?
    A. The specimen is transported immediately to the laboratory in a biohazard bag.
    B. The specimen appears hemolyzed.
    C. The specimen has a handwritten label.
    D. The specimen arrives to the laboratory with several other specimens that are STAT.

42. During venipunctue procedures that require blood specimens for multiple laboratory tests sometimes one additive/anticoagulant is carried over into the next tube. What effect can this have on laboratory testing?
    A. It has no effect if the tubes are filled to the correct level.
    B. It has no effect if the patient is normal and healthy.
    C. It can cause a violent chemical reaction that results in tube breakage.
    D. It can cause erroneous test results.

43. When collecting blood in an evacuated tube with an anticoagulant/additive, what is the importance of filling the tube until blood automatically stops entering the tube?
    A. It is important to maintain homeostasis.
    B. It prevents hemolysis.
    C. It promotes bleeding.
    D. It provides the correct blood-to-additive ratio.

44. How should the anticoagulant be mixed with a blood specimen in an evacuated tube?
    A. shaking the tube for 30 seconds
    B. centrifugation for 15 minutes
    C. mixing that occurs naturally as the specimen is transported
    D. gentle inversion of the specimen

45. Why is it important to monitor the daily amount of blood taken for venipunctures from pediatric or critically ill patients?
    A. It establishes an accurate glucose level.
    B. It helps determine the staffing level for the nursing unit.
    C. It helps reduce the incidence of iatrogenic anemia.
    D. It ensures that the tubes are labeled correctly.

46. TDM is useful for what type of analyses?
    A. hormone levels
    B. therapeutic drug levels
    C. thyroid diagnostics
    D. gastric analysis

47. The term "butterfly" refers to the:
    A. safety device on a needle
    B. evacuated collection tube
    C. winged infusion set
    D. a syringe

48. In a routine situation, how should a phlebotomist safely dispose of contaminated venipuncture supplies?
    A. Always use a puncture-resistant biohazard container.
    B. Take all contaminated supplies back to the laboratory.
    C. Transfer contaminated supplies to a biohazard plastic bag.
    D. Always use the wastebasket in the patient's hospital room.

Use the following scenario to refer to when answering Questions 49–51:

A health care worker entered a patient's room to collect blood specimens for the following tests: hematology cell counts, coagulation tests, blood cultures, and chemistry assays. The patient was an oncology patient and had scarring on many of her veins, had IVs in both forearms, and was diabetic. Laboratory notes indicated that blood should not be drawn from this patient's feet. Answer the following questions about this scenario.

49. Which site would be most suitable for blood collection?
    A. earlobe
    B. heel of the foot
    C. the posterior side of the hand or wrist
    D. the anterior surface of the wrist

50. What would be the preferred order of tube collection for these tests?
    A. blood cultures, coagulation, hematology, and chemistry
    B. blood cultures, chemistry, hematology, and coagulation
    C. hematology, coagulation, chemistry, and blood cultures
    D. coagulation, blood cultures, hematology, and chemistry

51. What measure could be taken to diminish the likelihood of complications when collecting blood for glucose, electrolytes, CBC, and PT?
    A. Use a butterfly system.
    B. Use a finger puncture.
    C. Decline to perform the venipuncture.
    D. Use a blood pressure cuff and tighten it more than usual to enhance pooling of the blood.

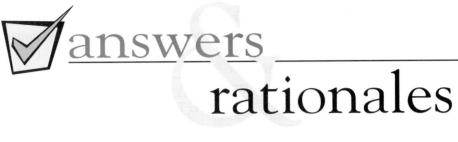

answers & rationales

1.

D. Use of gloves does not eliminate the need for hand hygiene, nor does good hand hygiene eliminate the need for gloves. (p. 307)

2.

B. Place gloves on after hands have been cleansed and in the presence of the patient. This gives both the patient and the phlebotomist a reassuring sense of a safety-conscious environment. (pp. 304–307)

3.

A. Normal skin is colonized with microorganisms; therefore, the transmission of pathogens by health care workers can occur easily. Adherence to hand-hygiene procedures has been shown to significantly reduce outbreaks of infections. (pp. 306–307)

4.

B. MRSA signifies methicillin-resistant *Staphylococcus aureus*. (p. 304)

5.

D. The safest way to identify an inpatient is a three-way match among the hospital identification bracelet, the test request that contains patient information, and the patient's verbal spelling of his or her name and birthdate. (p. 318)

6.

A. An inpatient identification armband must include the patient's first and last names and identification number. In addition, it may also include the patient's room number, bed assignment, and physician's name. (p. 319)

7.

D. If a hospitalized patient is semiconscious and/or has severe burns, he may not have an armband because it may be irritating to the burned areas of the skin. In this case the nurse in charge of the patient would be the best source for identifying the patient. The nurse's name should be documented. (pp. 317–318)

35.

A. Arteries do not feel like veins. They have thicker vessel walls, are more elastic, and pulsate. (p. 327)

36.

B. For patients who have had a mastectomy, lymph nodes are often removed from the same side. As a result swelling often occurs on the affected side of the body. Blood should not be withdrawn from the mastectomy side unless approved by a physician. However, the other arm's antecubital area should be considered first as an alternative site. (p. 327)

37.

B. In a venipuncture procedure, the needle should always be inserted into the skin with the bevel side upward and directly above a palpable, prominent vein. (p. 337)

38.

C. Patients do not like to be "stuck" more than once; however, the phlebotomist should try to locate a different, potentially good site and can try again. Phlebotomists should not make more than two venipuncture attempts on one patient. (p. 342)

39.

A. Winged infusion sets or butterfly needles are used for particularly difficult venipunctures. Young adult males usually have veins that are palpable and/or visible, so a winged infusion set would not be as useful compared to the other types of patients listed. (p. 342)

40.

A. Activating the safety device to cover the contaminated needle is the step that should be taken immediately after withdrawing the needle. This is usually done as the phlebotomist and/or patient presses gauze over the puncture site to contain bleeding. (p. 339)

41.

B. Specimens that are hemolyzed are often rejected for laboratory testing. (p. 354)

42.

D. If additives/anticoagulants are carried over into other test tubes, the test results can be erroneous. Many test results can be affected by accidental cross-contamination. It can be prevented by careful handling of the tubes, using the correct order of draw, and holding the tubes slightly downward during blood collection so that the additive stays at the bottom of the tube and is less likely to come into contact with the needle. (p. 347)

43.

D. The correct volume of blood in the specimen tube allows for the correct dilution ratio of additive to blood (blood-to-additive ratio). (p. 348)

44.

D. Gentle inversions of the specimen are needed to prevent the specimen from clotting. (pp. 339, 347)

45.

C. Processes that monitor the volume of blood taken from vulnerable patients (pediatric and critically ill) will reduce the incidence of iatrogenic anemia. (p. 351)

46.

B. Therapeutic drug monitoring or TDM is used to monitor correct dosage levels of the drug. (p. 355)

47.

C. The term "butterfly" refers to a winged infusion set. It actually refers to the small butterfly wing-like handles on the small needle apparatus. It is used to collect blood specimens from small or fragile veins. (pp. 340–341)

48.

A. Needles, syringes, tube holders, and other blood-letting devices should be discarded in a puncture-resistant biohazard container. (pp. 350–351)

49.

C. The posterior or dorsal side of the hand or wrist, below the IV site, could be used for venipuncture. (pp. 324–328)

50.

A. The preferred order of draw would be blood cultures, coagulation, hematology, and chemistry tubes. However, phlebotomists must follow the order of draw recommended by the manufacturers and their health care organizations. (pp. 345–346)

51.

A. Use of a butterfly system could diminish the likelihood of complications. Documentation of the circumstances surrounding this case would be warranted. (pp. 324–328)

CHAPTER

11 Capillary Blood Specimens

chapter objectives

Upon completion of Chapter 11, the learner is responsible for the following:

1. Describe the reasons for acquiring capillary blood specimens.
2. Explain why capillary blood from a skin puncture is different from blood taken by venipuncture and the impact on laboratory tests.
3. List the laboratory tests for which capillary specimens may be collected.
4. Identify the proper sites for performing a skin puncture procedure.
5. Explain why it is necessary to control the depth of the incision.
6. Describe the procedure for performing a skin puncture.
7. Describe the procedure for making blood smears.

DIRECTIONS Each of the questions or incomplete statements below is followed by four suggested answers or completions. Select one answer that is best in each case.

1. What effect does alcohol have on a skin puncture if it has not dried when the finger is punctured?
   A. prevents a round drop from forming
   B. facilitates making blood smears
   C. has a beneficial effect on laboratory tests
   D. provides an extra measure of sterility and reliability

2. The step that is not the same for a venipuncture and a finger-stick procedure is:
   A. patient identification
   B. hand hygiene
   C. angle of inserting the puncture device
   D. cleansing the site

3. Skin puncture techniques are most often used when:
   A. small amounts of blood are needed for testing or when the patient is a neonate
   B. the patient is normal but requires a large volume of blood for testing
   C. the patient is an athlete and needs a drug screen
   D. routine microbiology tests are needed

4. Which of the following steps would *not* be part of a finger-stick procedure?
   A. The patient's finger should be held firmly.
   B. The puncture should be made in one sharp, continuous movement.
   C. Pressure should be applied to the puncture site to expel the blood.
   D. The puncture site can be selected from anywhere on the skin.

5. Refer to the photos in Figure 11.1. In the first photo, which is/are the preferred skin puncture site(s)?
   A. thumb
   B. pointer finger
   C. third and fourth fingers
   D. pinky finger

FIGURE 11.1

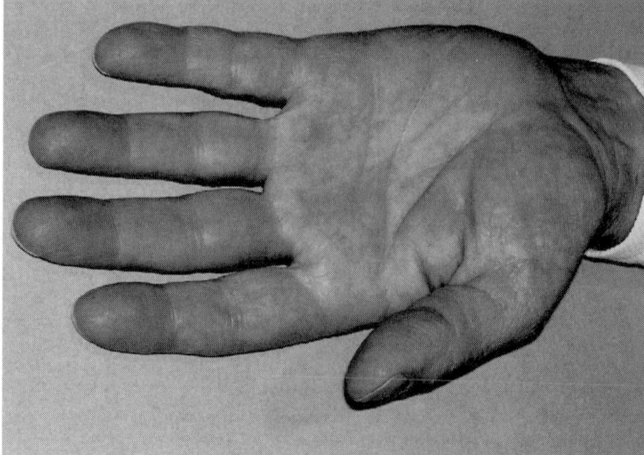

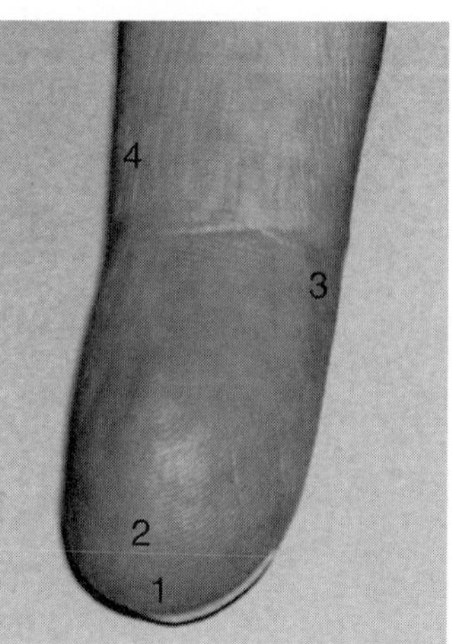

6. Refer to the second photo in Figure 11.1 to answer this question. Which of the following is the preferred region for a finger stick?
   A. the region of the finger labeled "1"
   B. the region of the finger labeled "2"
   C. the region of the finger labeled "3"
   D. the region of the finger labeled "4"

7. If a patient has had a mastectomy on his or her left side, which of the following sites would be best for a fingerstick?
   A. third or fourth left finger
   B. third or fourth right finger
   C. no skin puncture should be performed
   D. any finger of the left hand

8. Capillary blood acquired by skin puncture is composed of:
   A. mostly arterial blood
   B. mostly venous blood
   C. mostly intracellular and interstitial fluids
   D. arterial and venous blood and interstitial fluids

9. Fragile veins are most likely to be found in which type of patients?
   A. obese people
   B. people who do not exercise
   C. geriatric people
   D. teenagers

10. Capillary specimens are useful in which of the following situations?
   A. when veins are being saved for chemotherapy
   B. when a large volume of blood is needed for testing
   C. when blood cultures are being collected
   D. when hormone tests are being performed

11. What is interstitial fluid?
   A. synovial fluid
   B. capillary blood
   C. spinal fluid
   D. tissue fluid

12. Why is venipuncture more likely to cause problems for infants than adults?
   A. It is not more problematic for infants than adults.
   B. It makes children more likely to develop allergies.
   C. It increases the risks of anemia.
   D. It increases the risks of blood disorders.

13. Which reason explains how venipunctures can cause anemia?
   A. Too much blood is withdrawn.
   B. The procedure can be traumatic.
   C. The patient's anxiety can cause this problem.
   D. The cleansing procedure can cause this problem.

14. When and by whom should capillary specimens be labeled?
   A. immediately by the patient before the phlebotomist leaves
   B. immediately by the phlebotomist at the patient's side
   C. by the nurse when the phlebotomist exits the room
   D. by the laboratory staff when the phlebotomist logs in the patient's name

15. Which of the following conditions might have an adverse effect on the quality of a finger stick?
   A. the age of a patient
   B. the gender of a patient
   C. using the first drop of blood
   D. the presence of a wedding ring

16. Blood smears for the evaluation of cells must be made carefully. Which of the following features should not be present?
    A. one half of the slide being covered
    B. a feathered edge
    C. ridges and holes in the smear
    D. even, thin layer of blood

17. Why are manual, nonretractable lancets not recommended for use?
    A. Tissue fluids are more likely to be released.
    B. Blood is likely to be more arterialized.
    C. Manual, nonretractable lancets are indeed useful for geriatric patients.
    D. Depth of the puncture is harder to control.

18. Skin puncture samples are often used for which of the following situations?
    A. home testing
    B. blood cultures
    C. viral detection
    D. therapeutic drug levels

19. Which of the listed sequences is the best method for performing a finger stick?
    A. Squeeze the finger, cleanse the site, puncture the skin.
    B. Cleanse the site, squeeze the finger, puncture the skin, collect the first drop.
    C. Cleanse the site, puncture the skin, wipe the first drop, collect the sample.
    D. Apply tourniquet, puncture the skin, wipe the first drop, collect the sample.

20. Warming a site for skin puncture:
    A. increases blood pressure
    B. increases blood flow to the site
    C. relaxes the patient
    D. eliminates the need for a tourniquet

21. For most tests on capillary specimens, what should the phlebotomist do with the first drop of blood after a finger stick is performed?
    A. Use the first drop of blood for coagulation studies.
    B. Make a blood smear or slide.
    C. Wipe the first drop of blood off with gauze.
    D. Use the first drop of blood for hematology testing.

22. Which of the following facilitates site preparation for skin puncture?
    A. commercially available warming devices
    B. preheated tubes
    C. ice water
    D. gauze

23. What is the best angle for spreading a blood smear using two glass slides?
    A. 15 degrees
    B. 30 degrees
    C. 45 degrees
    D. 60 degrees

24. Normally, which of the following should be used to cleanse the site before skin puncture?
    A. isopropanol
    B. povidone-iodine
    C. diluted chlorox
    D. methanol

25. What is the average depth a skin puncture should be for an adult?
    A. 0.5–1.0 mm
    B. 2–3 mm
    C. 4–5 mm
    D. 5–7 mm

26. Excessive massaging or milking of the finger during a skin puncture procedure can cause:
    A. an adequate supply of blood for filling several capillary tubes
    B. increased venous blood flow to the puncture site
    C. hemolysis and contamination of the specimen with tissue fluids
    D. better results for glucose screening

27. Osteomyelitis is defined as:
    A. infection of the blood
    B. infection of the spinal fluid
    C. infection of the bone
    D. infection of the finger

28. How does a capillary tube fill with blood during a skin puncture procedure?
    A. Blood flows into the tube using suction from the collection device.
    B. Blood flows into the tube using the vacuum in the tube.
    C. Blood flows freely into the tube on contact.
    D. Gravity pulls the blood down into the tube.

29. In making a blood smear or slide, after the drop of blood has been spread across the glass slide, what is the next step?
    A. Gently blow on it to aid in drying.
    B. Hold it over a heating element to promote cellular adhesion to the glass.
    C. Add a drop of saline to the slide to preserve it.
    D. Allow it to air-dry.

30. What can happen if an EDTA microcollection tube is overfilled with blood?
    A. Clots may form in the tube.
    B. The patient is likely to faint.
    C. The tests will be falsely negative.
    D. The glucose test on the specimen will not be affected.

31. What can happen if an EDTA microcollection tube is underfilled?
    A. Clots may form in the tube.
    B. The patient is likely to faint.
    C. The tests will be falsely negative.
    D. Cell morphology will be altered.

32. Should clean glass capillary tubes be used routinely?
    A. No, because they break easily.
    B. No, because they hurt the patient.
    C. Yes, they are safe and effective.
    D. Yes, they are economical and easy to handle.

33. When is fasting an important consideration for collecting capillary specimens?
    A. It is only an important factor for collecting capillary specimens from the elderly.
    B. It is an important factor for collecting most capillary specimens.
    C. It is irrelevant and has no effect on capillary specimens.
    D. It is only an important factor when testing for glucose.

34. What effect does dehydration have on skin punctures?
    A. If a patient is dehydrated, it has no effect on the skin puncture.
    B. If a patient is dehydrated, bleeding may be more reduced so it is not recommended.
    C. If a patient is dehydrated, he or she is more likely to bleed excessively, so the phlebotomist should take extra precautions.
    D. If a patient is dehydrated, he or she is more likely to cough excessively during the procedure.

35. Why is the earlobe not a preferred site for skin puncture?
    A. It has more nerves than the other places on the body.
    B. It is close to the bone.
    C. It may cause anxiety due to the close proximity to the eyes.
    D. It is more easily bruised.

36. Which of the following is *not* a recommended site for skin puncture for pediatric cases?
    A. third finger
    B. fourth finger
    C. the pinkie finger
    D. heel of an infant

37. What is another term for PCV?
    A. pediatric cell volume
    B. hematocrit or packed cell volume
    C. pediatric cellular velocity
    D. hemoglobin or HGB value

38. Which of the following fingers has a pulse?
    A. pinky finger
    B. pointer finger
    C. middle finger
    D. thumb

39. Which of the following is the skin puncture device that is an alternative to a retractable lancet?
    A. radio frequency lancet
    B. scantag
    C. laser
    D. metallic clip

40. What type of lancet is most often recommended for skin puncture?
    A. nonretractable
    B. retractable
    C. puncture proof
    D. surgical lancet blade

41. The order of draw for filling microcollection tubes with capillary blood is:
    A. the same as for venipunctures
    B. not the same as for venipunctures
    C. the same as when using the butterfly method
    D. the same as for IV therapy

42. What is the appropriate order of filling microcollection tubes with capillary blood from a finger stick?
    A. EDTA specimen for hematology tests, other tubes with additives, nonadditive tubes
    B. additive tubes, then nonadditive tubes
    C. coagulation tubes, then nonadditive tubes
    D. EDTA tubes should always be filled last after other tubes have been filled

43. Capillary blood cannot be used for which of the following test analyses?
    A. glucose and lactose
    B. blood cultures and coagulation studies
    C. cholesterol screening tests
    D. blood gases

44. How should used lancets be disposed?
    A. puncture-proof trash can
    B. puncture-proof biohazard sharps container
    C. biohazard bag along with contaminated gauze
    D. a container with alcohol

45. Which statement describes a cyanotic finger?
    A. bluish in color due to insufficient oxygen
    B. yellow in color due to liver failure
    C. green in color due to infection
    D. red and swollen

46. During a skin puncture procedure, how should the cut be oriented on the finger?
    A. on a diagonal
    B. parallel to the fingerprint lines
    C. across the fingerprint lines
    D. It doesn't matter how the lancet is positioned, it is done automatically.

47. After a skin puncture procedure, where should the phlebotomist dispose of contaminated gloves?
    A. Contaminated gloves should be disposed of in the trash can located at the patient's bedside.
    B. They should be disposed of in a biohazard container near the procedure area.
    C. They should be transported to the laboratory and disposed of with other lab trash.
    D. Gloves should be taken to the nursing station for proper disposal.

48. How should the phlebotomist treat a microcollection tube with additives once the blood specimen is taken?
    A. It should be shaken vigorously.
    B. It should be frozen.
    C. It should be mixed gently.
    D. It should be placed in a warm location.

49. Air bubbles in microcollection tubes can do which of the following?
    A. assist in blood flow
    B. keep the blood from spilling out of the tube
    C. cause delayed clotting
    D. cause erroneous results

50. What procedure is needed when collecting capillary blood for blood gases?
    A. cooling the puncture site
    B. warming the puncture site
    C. sticking deeper into the skin
    D. using a special arterial lancet

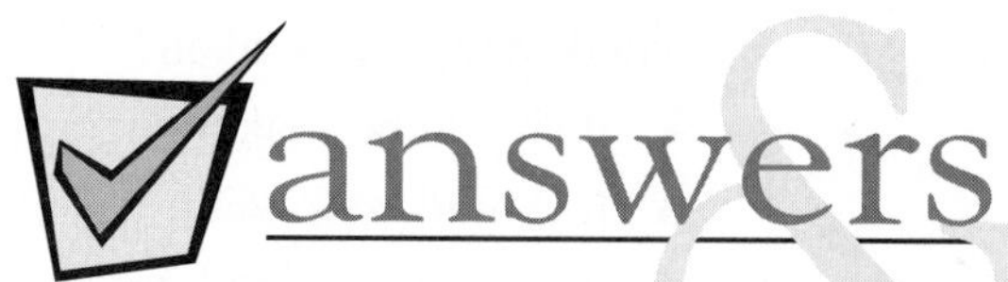

answers & rationales

1.

A. If alcohol does not dry prior to a skin puncture, the residual alcohol prevents round drops of blood from forming. (p. 372)

2.

C. The angle of inserting the puncture device is different for venipuncture needles and skin puncture devices. Skin puncture devices should be used according to the manufacturer's instructions, but for most types, the device is positioned directly on the clean puncture site and not at an angle. Refer to procedure 11.1. (p. 372)

3.

A. Skin puncture techniques are most often used when small amounts of blood are needed for testing, for neonates, or when other complications warrant it. (p. 364)

4.

D. The puncture should be done in one sharp, continuous movement on the third or fourth fingers in designated areas. (p. 369)

5.

C. The preferred puncture sites are the third or fourth fingers. (p. 369)

6.

B. The fleshy portion of the finger (third or fourth fingers), not the fingertip, should be punctured. This is most closely represented by the region labeled "2." (p. 369)

7.

B. As mentioned when discussing venipunctures, a patient who has had a mastectomy on one side has excess lymph fluid on that side; thus, any blood specimen should be collected on the other side when possible. (p. 369)

8.

D. Capillary blood is a combination of blood from arteries, veins, capillaries, and interstitial fluids. (p. 365)

9.

C. Fragile veins are often found in geriatric patients. (p. 364)

10.

A. Capillary specimens are useful when veins are being saved for chemotherapy in oncology patients. (p. 364)

11.

D. Interstitial fluid is tissue fluid. (p. 364)

12.

C. Venipunctures are more problematic for infants because of the increased risk of complications such as iatrogenic anemia. Since the total blood volume of infants is small, a blood specimen taken by venipuncture can remove a significant portion of their total blood volume and cause anemia. (p. 364)

13.

A. When too much blood is withdrawn from a small child or infant, the blood volume may be significantly reduced. (p. 364)

14.

B. Specimens should be labeled immediately after collection by the phlebotomist. (p. 378)

15.

C. Using the first drop of blood can have an adverse effect on a skin puncture specimen because it may be diluted with interstitial fluids, thus causing erroneous test results. However, some point-of-care instruments do not require this step, so it is important to follow the manufacturer's instructions. (p. 372)

16.

C. No ridges, lines, or holes should be present on a blood smear. (p. 377)

17.

D. Use of manual, nonretractable lancets is not recommended because the depth of the puncture is harder to control. (p. 374)

18.

A. Skin puncture specimens can be useful for many home testing applications. They are also used for various screening tests and/or point-of-care procedures. (p. 364)

19.

C. The best procedure would be to cleanse the site, puncture the skin, wipe the first drop (unless otherwise required), and collect the specimen. (pp. 365–366)

20.

B. Warming the site for a skin puncture procedure increases blood flow to the area. (p. 370)

21.

C. For most tests on capillary blood specimens, the first drop of blood expelled after the puncture should be wiped off. (p. 371)

22.

A. Commercially available warming devices can facilitate site preparation. (p. 370)

23.

B. The best angle for spreading a blood smear using two slides is approximately 30 degrees. (p. 377)

24.

A. Isopropanol should be used to cleanse the site before skin puncture. (p. 372)

25.

B. The average depth for a skin puncture should be 2–3 mm for an adult; this avoids hitting the bone. (p. 373)

26.

C. Excessive milking and massaging of the finger can cause hemolysis and contamination of the specimen with tissue fluids. (p. 373)

27.

C. Osteomyelitis is defined as inflammation and infection of the bone. (p. 374)

28.

C. Blood flows freely into the capillary tube on contact; this is called capillary action. (p. 372)

29.

D. Blood smears should be allowed to air-dry. (p. 377)

30.

A. Overfilling an EDTA tube can cause clot formation and render the specimen unacceptable. (p. 375)

31.

D. The ratio of EDTA to blood will be inaccurate if the EDTA tube is underfilled and it may alter the WBC morphology. (p. 375)

32.

A. Unless they are specially designed to reduce breakage, glass capillary tubes should not be routinely used. (p. 368)

33.

B. Fasting status is important for collecting most types of blood specimens. (pp. 367, 371)

34.

B. If a patient is dehydrated, bleeding after the puncture will be reduced, so a skin puncture is not recommended. If the patient drinks a glass of water to rehydrate himself or herself and rests for a period of time, then the fingers can be reevaluated for a puncture. (p. 364)

35.

C. Use of the earlobe for skin puncture is still in practice by some phlebotomists; however, it is not preferred due to possible interference with other body piercings, and the close proximity to the eyes may cause undue anxiety and flinching during the procedure. (p. 369)

36.

C. The pinkie finger is not recommended because the tissue of this finger is considerably thinner than that of the others, and there is a risk of hitting the bone. (p. 369)

37.

B. Hematocrit or packed cell volume is another term for PCV. (p. 375)

38.

D. The thumb has a pulse. (p. 369)

39.

C. A laser device is an acceptable skin puncture device for collecting capillary specimens. (p. 373)

40.

B. Retractable puncture devices are recommended for skin puncture procedures. (p. 373)

41.

B. The order of draw for filling tubes with capillary blood is not the same as for venipuncture tubes. (p. 374)

42.

A. The correct order of filling microcollection tubes with capillary blood is EDTA tubes for hematology tests, other tubes with additives, and last, nonadditive tubes. (p. 375)

43.

B. Blood cultures and coagulation studies should not be performed using capillary blood specimens. (p. 364)

44.

B. Lancets should be disposed of in a puncture-proof biohazard sharps container. (p. 378)

45.

A. A cyanotic finger is bluish in color due to insufficient oxygen. (p. 371)

46.

C. During a skin puncture or finger stick, the cut should be oriented across or perpendicular to the ridges of the fingerprint grooves. (p. 372)

47.

B. Gloves should be disposed of in a biohazard container near the procedure area. (p. 373)

48.

C. Specimens should be gently inverted to mix additives with the blood specimen. (p. 373)

49.

D. Air bubbles in capillary blood specimen tubes can cause erroneous laboratory results. (p. 373)

50.

B. Warming the site prior to capillary blood gases will increase arterial blood flow to the area. (p. 378)

CHAPTER

12 Specimen Handling, Transportation, and Processing

chapter objectives

Upon completion of Chapter 12, the learner is responsible for the following:

1. Describe at least three sources of preexamination error that can occur during blood specimen handling.
2. Describe at least three sources of preexamination error that can occur during blood specimen transportation.
3. Describe at least three sources of preexamination error that can occur during specimen processing or storage.
4. Name three methods commonly used to transport specimens.

DIRECTIONS Each of the questions or incomplete statements below is followed by four suggested answers or completions. Select one answer that is best in each case.

1. When does a phlebotomist's job end in regard to handling a blood specimen?
   A. when the phlebotomist leaves the patient after the venipuncture
   B. when all the tubes are labeled
   C. when the specimen is delivered to the laboratory
   D. when the specimen is transported, processed, and tested

2. Once blood has been added to an evacuated tube containing additives, how soon should it be mixed?
   A. immediately
   B. within 10 minutes
   C. 11–30 minutes
   D. 30–60 minutes

3. Which of the following refers to the time it takes for a specimen to be ordered, collected, transported, processed, analyzed, and reported?
   A. transcription time
   B. error reduction time
   C. turnaround time
   D. reporting time

4. The phlebotomist has the greatest impact on which phase of laboratory testing?
   A. postanalytic phase
   B. preanalytic phase
   C. analytic phase
   D. specimen processing

5. Which of the following variables represents a preanalytic variable that might affect laboratory testing results?
   A. not wearing a laboratory coat
   B. reporting laboratory test results to the nurse
   C. the patient eating a hearty breakfast
   D. the specimen being tested on a calibrated instrument

6. What is a likely result if a specimen tube containing additives is not mixed correctly?
   A. a higher risk of infections
   B. more patient discomfort
   C. tiny clots may form within the tube
   D. a greater chance for breakage in the centrifuge

7. To protect the phlebotomist or other health care workers, what container should be used to transport blood specimens?
   A. the phlebotomist's clean lab coat pockets
   B. a leakproof biohazard bag
   C. an opaque, plastic, color-coded box
   D. a four-sided biohazard waste container

8. Glycolytic action refers to which of the following?
   A. a serious medical crisis
   B. cellular morphology
   C. clotting factors
   D. breakdown of glucose

9. What effect will rough handling and transportation delays likely have on coagulation test results?
   A. no significant changes
   B. platelet activation and shortened clotting times
   C. increased cholesterol factors
   D. increased WBC counts

10. A phlebotomist was asked by a patient to let him or her see the final labeled blood specimen. What is the most appropriate course of action for the phlebotomist?
    A. Allow the patient to check the labels on the blood specimen.
    B. Do not allow the patient to check the labels.
    C. Allow the patient to mix the specimen.
    D. Explain to the patient that specimens now belong to the laboratory.

11. Why is the speed of delivery of specimens especially important for blood gas analyses?
    A. The patients needing this test are usually pediatric patients.
    B. Blood gases are light sensitive.
    C. Blood gases are motion sensitive.
    D. Gases from the specimen can easily leak out over time.

12. Which of the following agencies offers recommendations for transport and handling of blood specimens for clinical laboratory testing?
    A. The Joint Commission
    B. CLSI
    C. ASCP
    D. NPA

13. What additional equipment item is necessary when transporting a specimen at 37°C?
    A. a pocket blood analyzer for cholesterol
    B. a heat source or heat block
    C. a chilled source or ice block
    D. a radio frequency identification (RFID) receiver

14. Cooling a blood specimen causes which of the following to occur?
    A. slowing down of metabolic processes
    B. hemolysis
    C. increasing bacterial reproduction
    D. poor separation during centrifugation

15. What is the likely consequence of inadequate mixing of a gel separation tube?
    A. There should be no harmful consequence.
    B. The gel will stick to the sides of the tube.
    C. Blood clotting may be incomplete.
    D. Chemical breakdown of the specimen will occur.

16. As a general rule of thumb, blood specimens should be transported to the laboratory for testing within which of the following time periods to prevent erroneous test results?
    A. 8 hours
    B. 6 hours
    C. 4 hours
    D. as soon as possible

17. What is the preferred time period for transporting blood specimens for coagulation testing?
    A. 6–8 hours
    B. 4–6 hours
    C. 2–4 hours
    D. less than 1 hour

18. Approximately how long does it take for a normal blood specimen to clot at room temperature?
   A. 1–2 minutes
   B. 5–10 minutes
   C. 30–60 minutes
   D. about 2 hours

19. The term "thermolabile" refers to a trait of some chemical constituents that are tested in blood specimens. What does it mean?
   A. Constituents are affected by temperature.
   B. Constituents are affected by light.
   C. Constituents are affected by the method of draw.
   D. Constituents are affected by the time of day that the specimen is drawn.

20. Excessive agitation of a specimen is likely to cause which of the following conditions?
   A. thorough mixing of the anticoagulant with the blood
   B. warming of the specimen
   C. chilling of the specimen
   D. hemolysis in the specimen

21. Some specimens are wrapped in aluminum foil during transportation. What purpose does this serve?
   A. keeps the specimen warm
   B. keeps the specimen cool
   C. protects the specimen from light
   D. protects the specimen from unnecessary agitation

22. Hemolyzed specimens cause which of the following?
   A. chemical interference with lab assays
   B. warming of the specimen
   C. cooling of the specimen
   D. centrifugation interference

23. If a blood specimen has a separation device, how many times should it be centrifuged?
   A. maximum of eight times
   B. five to seven times
   C. two to four times
   D. only one time

24. If the laboratory must save separated serum or plasma for testing later, how would most specimens be stored after 8 hours?
   A. at 22°C
   B. at 2–8°C
   C. in a frost-free freezer section of a refrigerator
   D. at or below –20°C

25. What purpose does an amber-colored biohazard bag serve?
   A. prevents lysing of the RBCs
   B. prevents lysing of the WBCs
   C. prevents breakdown of glucose
   D. prevents degradation of photosensitive substances

26. Why might one use an airtight container with icy water to transport an arterial specimen for blood gas analysis?
   A. It decreases the loss of gases from the specimen.
   B. It promotes coagulation.
   C. It aids in the instrumentation phase of the testing process.
   D. It increases the oxygen content in the specimen.

27. Assays that require a chilled specimen do *not* include which of the following?
   A. gastrin, ammonia, and lactic acid
   B. renin, catecholamine, and parathyroid hormone determinations

C. blood gases
D. blood cultures

28. To chill a blood specimen as it is transported, the health care worker should use:
A. tepid water
B. a small freezer unit
C. icy water or commercial cool pack
D. frozen blocks of ice

29. Specimens that require protection from light include those for:
A. CBC, diff, and platelet counts
B. PT and PTTs
C. bilirubin and some vitamins
D. glucose and cholesterol

30. Specimens that require warming to body temperature are those for:
A. CBC, diff, and platelet counts
B. PT and PTTs
C. bilirubin and some vitamins
D. cold agglutinins and cryofibrinogen

31. Most laboratories require that primary specimen tubes be placed in which of the following during transportation?
A. biohazard box
B. leakproof plastic bag
C. aluminum foil
D. icy water

32. Why should blood and urine specimens for microbiological culture be transported to the laboratory quickly?
A. Blood cells will not rupture.
B. It will improve the likelihood of detecting the presence of drugs.
C. It will reduce the time for detecting pathogens.
D. It will avoid excessive exposure to light.

33. One of the most efficient and safest methods of specimen transportation in a large health care organization is:
A. hand-carrying the specimen
B. pneumatic tube systems
C. clear biohazard carts
D. email for specimens

34. Laboratory reports containing test results should go through which of the following protocols?
A. Release results immediately upon completion of the testing process.
B. Confirm results, date the release of results, and forward a permanent copy to the clinical record.
C. Call the results to a physician.
D. Fax the results immediately to the patient.

35. What effect would a patient's heparin therapy have on processing the specimen?
A. It will lengthen clotting time.
B. It will cause photosensitivity.
C. It will increase centrifugation time.
D. It will have no effect.

36. In designing a report form for laboratory results (either electronic or paper version), which one of the listed elements could be omitted?
A. patient and physician identification
B. date and time of collection
C. reference ranges
D. patient and physician addresses

36.

D. The addresses of patient and physician are not usually needed on a laboratory test report. (pp. 397–398)

37.

D. Gel and nongel devices form a barrier between the serum/plasma and the blood clot/cells during centrifugation. Each device has a particular viscosity and specific gravity that is between the weights of the serum/plasma and the cells. (p. 393)

38.

A. Blood specimens can be transported in many pneumatic tube systems if they are contained in a leakproof biohazard bag or container surrounded by shock-absorbing padding. (p. 391)

39.

C. Blood specimens should be balanced in a centrifuge. This means that each tube should have a corresponding tube directly across from it in the centrifuge holder. Refer to Figure 12.6. (p. 393)

40.

B. An aliquot is a portion of the blood specimen that has been subdivided so that it can be tested in another location or another instrument in the laboratory. The same identification information or code should be placed on each aliquot specimen so that it can be traced back to that individual original specimen when necessary. (p. 394)

41.

C. Packaging for blood specimens being shipped by air must contain an inner/primary package surrounded by an outer/secondary container. (p. 396)

42.

A. Breakage of a specimen during transportation in a pneumatic tube is an example of a preanalytical error due to a transportation variable. It can be prevented by careful packaging of the specimen prior to sending it. (p. 391)

43.

D. The primary or inner package used for shipping biohazardous specimens by air should be watertight, and each specimen tube should be individually wrapped. (p. 396)

44.

D. The secondary or outer package required for shipping biohazardous specimens by air should also be watertight and contain absorbent material capable of absorbing all contents of the primary receptacle. (p. 396)

45.

B. Critical value, sometimes referred to as panic value, is a test result that may be life-threatening. (p. 399)

46–48.

C, B, A. This short case involves lessons on several topics, including communication skills and time management (handled in earlier chapters), specimen handling, and processing. This describes a somewhat stressful environment where Mary decided to take some shortcuts that were not completely appropriate. First, as was mentioned in earlier chapters, the phone should be answered on the first or second ring. Secondly, she likely loaded the specimens into the centrifuge in an unbalanced orientation that may cause breakage or insufficient cell separation. Thirdly, she shortened the centrifugation time, which is a critical parameter in achieving an adequate separation and barrier placement if present, and ultimately could cause some analytical interference. And fourth, she removed the caps from the tubes prior to centrifugation, which caused a significant safety risk for contamination of the inside of the centrifuge. Cleaning up after a spill would be hazardous and time consuming, as well as causing the need for re-collecting the patient. All actions could have been prevented if she had followed appropriate protocols. (pp. 392–393)

49–50.

D, B. General packaging requirements for infectious substances, or diagnostic specimens, are important for safety and compliance issues. Acceptable and leakproof primary and secondary containers should be used, and the secondary container should be of sufficient strength to withstand a stacking test and a drop test. Also, a refrigerant should be secured outside the secondary container, with a support to contain any condensation or refrigerant even after it has evaporated, etc. If dry ice is used, the outer packaging must allow for the release of CO_2 gas. (pp. 396–397)

CHAPTER

13 Pediatric and Geriatric Procedures

chapter objectives

Upon completion of Chapter 13, the learner is responsible for the following:

1. Describe fears or concerns that children in different developmental stages might have toward the blood collection process.
2. List suggestions that might be appropriate for parental and health care worker behavior during a venipuncture or skin puncture.
3. Identify puncture sites for a heel stick on an infant, and describe the procedure.
4. Describe the venipuncture sites for infants and young children.
5. Discuss the types of equipment and supplies that must be used during microcollection and venipuncture of infants and children.
6. Explain the special precautions and types of equipment needed to collect capillary blood gases.
7. Describe the procedure for specimen collection for neonatal screening.

8. Define five physical and/or emotional changes that are associated with the aging process.
9. Describe how a health care worker should react to physical and emotional changes associated with the elderly.

DIRECTIONS

Each of the questions or incomplete statements below is followed by four suggested answers or completions. Select one answer that is best in each case.

1. Warming the infant's heel prior to blood collection provides which of the following benefits?
   A. hastens hemostasis
   B. increases the blood flow
   C. causes the capillary blood to become similar to venous blood for better testing purposes
   D. decreases the possibility of abnormal coagulation

2. To be effective, EMLA must be applied at least how long before venipuncture?
   A. 10 minutes
   B. 20 minutes
   C. 45 minutes
   D. 1 hour

3. When performing skin punctures, the phlebotomist needs to collect chemistry specimens:
   A. first
   B. second
   C. third
   D. fourth

4. Which is *not* a preferred site on the heel for a heel stick?
   A. medial aspect
   B. lateral aspect
   C. central area
   D. lateral section of the plantar surface

5. In a child, the distance from the skin surface to the bone or cartilage in the third finger is between:
   A. 0.85 and 1.5 mm
   B. 1.5 and 2.4 mm
   C. 2.4 and 3.1 mm
   D. 3.1 and 3.4 mm

6. Which of the following is *not* a normal acceptable intervention to alleviate pain when performing venipuncture on an infant?
   A. EMLA cream
   B. oral sucrose
   C. lidocaine injection
   D. pacifier

7. As depicted in Figure 13.1, what procedure is being used related to needlestick insertion?
   A. A cream is being applied to decrease the possibility of severe bleeding from blood collection.
   B. An anesthetic cream is being applied to decrease needlestick pain.
   C. An anesthetic cream is being applied to alleviate the latex reaction that occurred after a Band-Aid was applied over the needlestick insertion.
   D. A cream is being applied prior to blood collection since the patient is allergic to metal in needles.

FIGURE 13.1

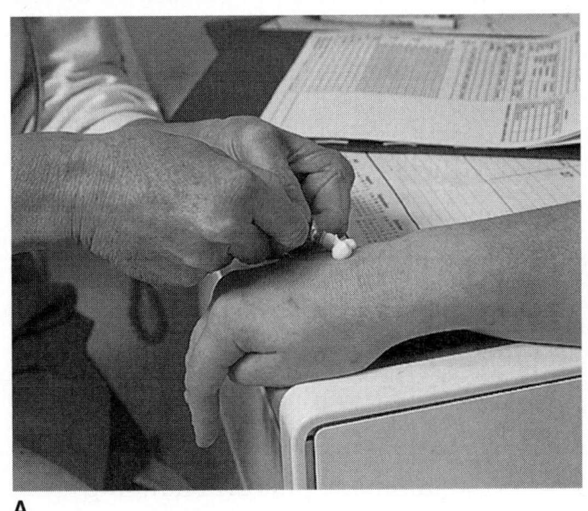

A

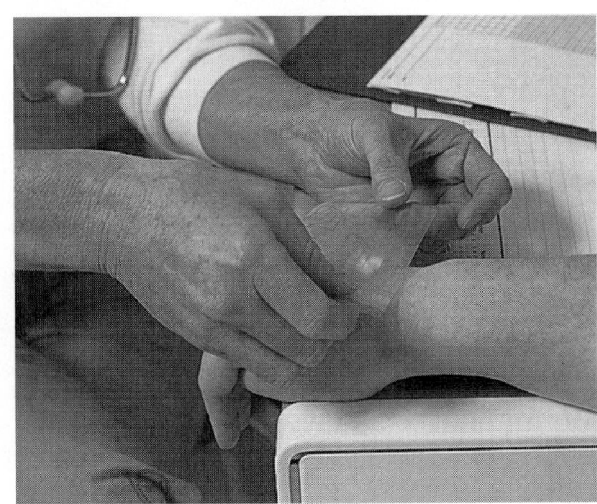

B

8. After a capillary blood gas collection, pressure should be applied over the skin puncture site with a dry gauze sponge:
   A. for 20–30 seconds
   B. for 30–60 seconds
   C. for 1/2–1 1/2 minutes
   D. until the bleeding stops

9. The venipuncture technique for infants as shown in Figure 13.2 requires the positioning of the needle at what degree angle over the vein for a correct, safe blood collection?
   A. 45 degree
   B. 30 degree
   C. 25 degree
   D. 15 degree

FIGURE 13.2

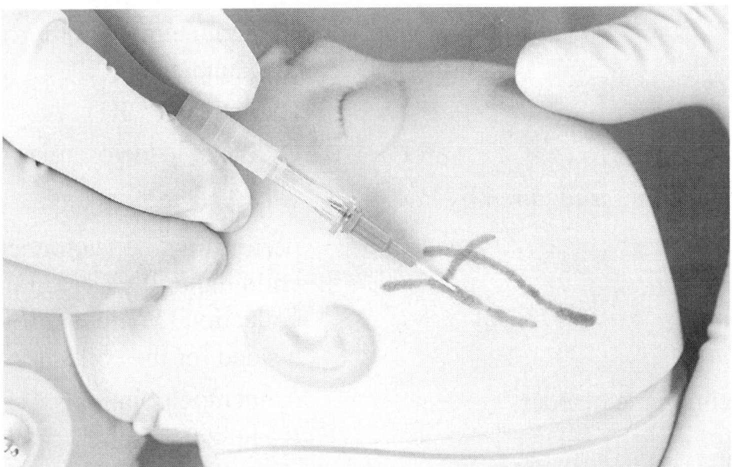

10. When a skin puncture is performed on an infant or a child, which of the following specimens is collected first?
    A. blood bank specimens
    B. chemistry specimens
    C. clinical immunology specimens
    D. hematology specimens

11. A sterile gauze sponge should be pressed against the infant's heel after skin puncture for blood collection in order to:
    A. avoid increased coagulation
    B. avoid a hematoma
    C. increase RBCs to the site
    D. decrease calcium

12. A child in what age group would perceive pain from a needlestick as a punishment for bad behavior?
    A. 1 year old
    B. 3–5 years old
    C. 6–10 years old
    D. 11–15 years old

13. The total blood volume of a premature infant is calculated by multiplying weight in kilograms by:
    A. 115 mL/kg
    B. 80–110 mL/kg
    C. 75–100 mL/kg
    D. 70 mL/kg

14. Neonatal blood screening is required by law to test for:
    A. hypoadrenalism
    B. hypothyroidism
    C. spina bifida
    D. congenital neurogenic bladder anomaly

15. What age group is embarrassed to show fear when venipuncture is performed on them?
    A. 1–3 years old
    B. 3–5 years old
    C. 6–12 years old
    D. 13–17 years old

16. When performing skin puncture on an infant or child, the designated order of draw for hematology specimens occurs for which of the following reasons?
    A. to minimize increased RBCs in the microcollection containers
    B. to minimize platelet clumping
    C. to increase WBCs and RBCs in the containers for blood cell counts
    D. to maintain the proper blood pH

17. If a venipuncture needs to be performed on a child younger than 2 years of age, the recommended site is:
    A. cephalic vein
    B. axillary vein
    C. medial wrist vein
    D. basilic vein

18. Newborns are routinely screened through blood analysis for which of the following genetic and metabolic defects?
    A. diabetes, congenital hypothyroidism
    B. congenital hypothyroidism, obstructive jaundice
    C. diabetes, PKU
    D. PKU, galactosemia

19. Which of the following is a reason for performing the venipuncture procedure on a child rather than a skin puncture for blood collection? Venipuncture on a child is needed for the collection of specimens for:
    A. hemoglobin
    B. blood cultures

C. hematocrit
D. cholesterol

20. A complication that can occur from a neonatal heel stick is:
    A. PKU
    B. congenital adrenal hyperplasia
    C. osteomyelitis
    D. toxoplasmosis

21. If 20 mL of blood is collected from a premature infant (weighing 4.0 kg) over a 2-day period, approximately what percentage of the baby's total blood volume is that?
    A. 1%
    B. 4%
    C. 8%
    D. 20%

22. Figure 13.3 shows what vein to be used for blood collection in children?
    A. median cubital vein
    B. dorsal vein
    C. femoral vein
    D. anterior tibial vein

23. A latex-free tourniquet is absolutely necessary for a child with:
    A. chicken pox
    B. strep throat
    C. PKU
    D. spina bifida

24. Which of the following is needed for blood collection by skin puncture on an infant?
    A. puncture-resistant sharps container
    B. Eclipse safety needle
    C. purple-topped evacuated tube
    D. Velcro-type tourniquet

FIGURE 13.3

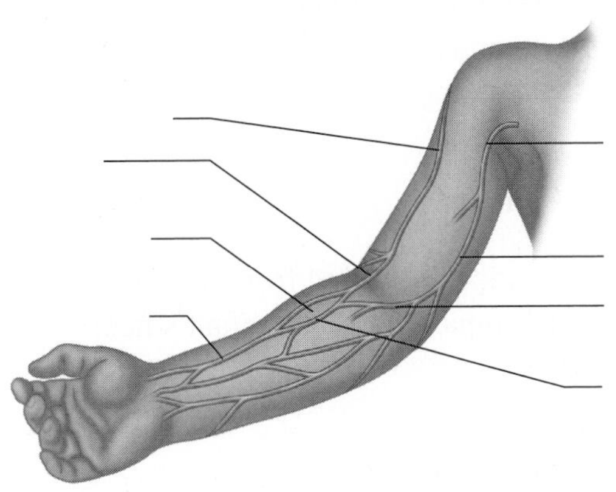

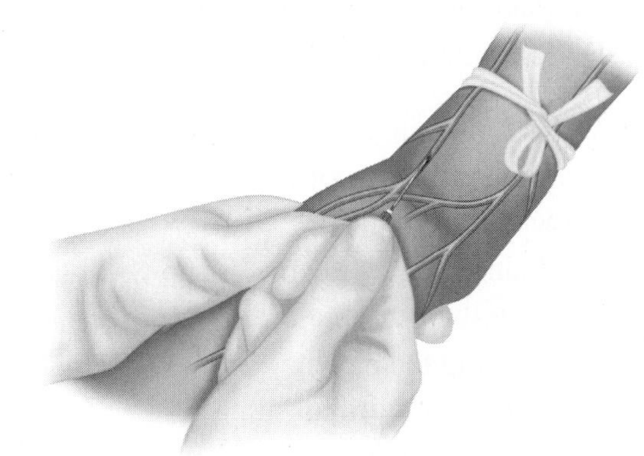

25. What needle gauge size is required for scalp vein venipuncture of an infant?
    A. 17
    B. 19
    C. 21
    D. 23

26. In the collection of blood cultures from infants, which of the following is the preferred antiseptic to use prior to blood collection?
    A. 70% isopropyl alcohol
    B. chlorhexidine gluconate
    C. iodine
    D. Betadine

27. To prewarm the infant's heel for blood collection, it is best to prewarm the site for:
    A. 30 seconds
    B. 1–2 minutes
    C. 3–5 minutes
    D. 5–8 minutes

28. Complications resulting from multiple deep skin punctures on an infant's heel include:
    A. hepatitis
    B. osteomyelitis
    C. pneumonia
    D. HIV infection

29. When collecting blood from a saline lock on a child, the blood collector must check the patency of the line by:
    A. disinfecting the catheter cap with alcohol or iodine solution
    B. flushing the catheter cap with a small amount of normal saline
    C. injecting slowly the heparinized flush solution
    D. flushing the catheter cap with a small amount of glucose solution

30. For the performance of a heel stick on an infant, the infant should be positioned in the:
    A. lateral position
    B. supine position
    C. prone position
    D. recovery position

31. Blood spot testing for neonatal screening is performed before the newborn is:
    A. 24 hours old
    B. 36 hours old
    C. 48 hours old
    D. 72 hours old

32. Blood collection for neonatal screening to detect metabolic and genetic abnormalities occurs on blood collected from:
    A. the infant's scalp vein
    B. the infant's median cubital vein
    C. the infant's lateral plantar surface of the heel
    D. the infant's dorsal vein

33. Figure 13.4 shows blood being collected for:
    A. blood gases
    B. hematology testing
    C. neonatal metabolic screening
    D. chemistry screening

34. The best location for performing a phlebotomy on a hospitalized child is:
    A. at the bedside in a chair
    B. in a playroom
    C. in a treatment room
    D. in his or her bed

35. After the blood is collected from the newborn for PKU testing, the card must dry in a horizontal position for a minimum of:
    A. 30 minutes
    B. 1 hour
    C. 2 hours
    D. 4 hours

FIGURE 13.4 Wadsworth Center, New York State Department of Health.

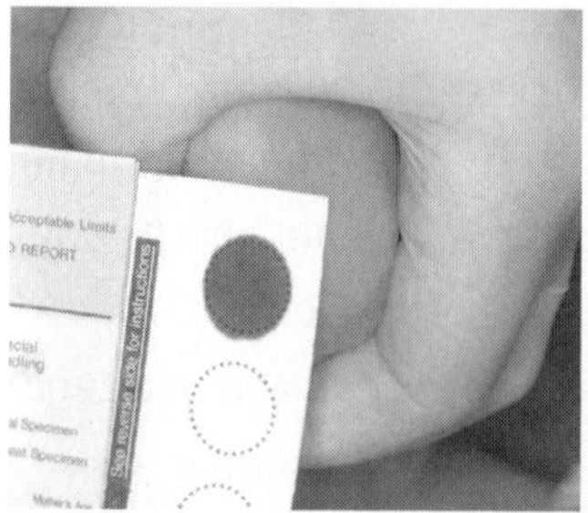

36. Which of the following is an emotional factor associated with geriatric patients?
    A. anemia
    B. cystic fibrosis
    C. depression
    D. PKU

37. The optimal depth of a finger stick in a child is:
    A. greater than 3.0 mm
    B. less than 0.5 mm
    C. less than 3.0 mm
    D. less than 2.0 mm

38. To collect blood from IV lines in a hospitalized child, which of the following is needed for a safe method to avoid a needlestick injury?
    A. transfer device for transferring blood into vacuum tubes
    B. butterfly needle for insertion into the IV line
    C. 21-gauge needle
    D. safety lancet

39. Why does OSHA mandate that latex or silicone membrane ports be used on CVCs?
    A. They are slippery and thus the needle can enter more easily into the port for blood collection.
    B. These ports can be easily disinfected before entry for blood collection.
    C. These ports allow penetration with a needless access device.
    D. Both B and C are correct.

40. When performing venipuncture on a child's arm, the recommended needle gauge size is:
    A. 17
    B. 19
    C. 23
    D. 25

41. Which is the preferred site for a heel stick?
    A. anteromedial aspect
    B. posterior curve
    C. medial or lateral aspect
    D. a previous puncture site

42. A 10-mL blood sample taken from a premature or newborn infant is equivalent to what percent of the infant's total blood volume?
    A. 1–2%
    B. 3–4%
    C. 5–10%
    D. 10–15%

43. A commonly inherited disease that is detected through the mandatory neonatal blood screening process is:
    A. anemia
    B. spina bifida
    C. neurogenic bladder abnormality
    D. PKU

44. A premature infant weighing 2.0 kilograms has what total blood volume?
    A. 130 mL
    B. 215 mL
    C. 230 mL
    D. 430 mL

45. Venipuncture in children is indicated for which of the following laboratory tests?
    A. hemoglobin
    B. blood cultures
    C. WBC
    D. glucose

46. When collecting blood from a child's long-term CVC, what size syringe should be used?
    A. 1 mL
    B. 3 mL
    C. 5 mL
    D. 10 mL

47. EMLA is sometimes used for pediatric venipuncture procedures. EMLA is a:
    A. local anesthetic applied with a small needle to the child's arm before venipuncture
    B. topical anesthetic applied to the child's arm before venipuncture
    C. topical lotion applied to the child's arm after venipuncture to stop bleeding at the venipuncture site
    D. topical lotion applied to the child's arm before venipuncture to assist the phlebotomist in finding a vein

48. For a 3-year-old child, which of the following skin puncture sites is most frequently used for blood collection?
    A. medial section of the bottom of the heel
    B. lateral section of the bottom of the heel
    C. palmar surface of the tip of the thumb
    D. palmar surface of the tip of the fourth finger

49. Which of the following is an acceptable intervention to alleviate pain during venipuncture on a child?
    A. lidocaine
    B. sucrose nipple
    C. ice pack
    D. EMLA

50. The angle of the needle for a pediatric venipuncture should be:
    A. 30 degrees or less with the skin surface
    B. 45 degrees or less with the skin surface
    C. 55 degrees or less with the skin surface
    D. 60 degrees or less with the skin surface

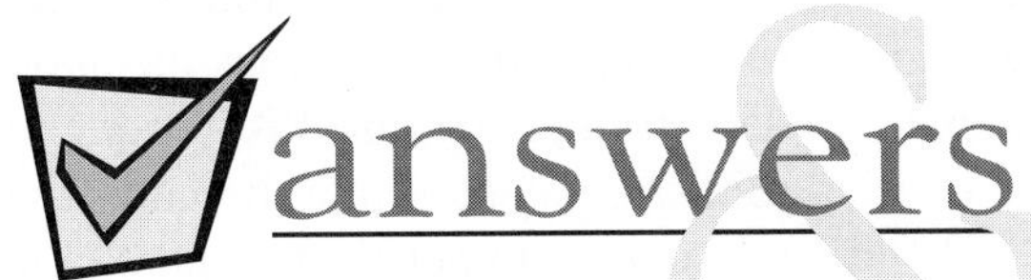

answers & rationales

1.

B. Prewarming the infant's heel prior to blood collection increases the blood flow. (p. 418)

2.

D. For optimal effectiveness, EMLA should be applied at least 1 hour before venipuncture. (p. 413)

3.

B. When performing skin punctures, the phlebotomist needs to collect the hematology specimens first, then the chemistry specimens with additives. (p. 416)

4.

C. The medial or most lateral section of the plantar surface of the heel should be used, *not* the central area. (p. 416)

5.

B. In a child, the distance from the skin surface to the bone or cartilage in the third finger is between 1.5 and 2.4 mm. Thus, an automatic skin puncture device should not exceed 2.0 mm in small children. (p. 428)

6.

C. Using EMLA cream, oral sucrose, and a pacifier and swaddling are the normal acceptable methods to alleviate pain from venipuncture in an infant. (pp. 413–414)

7.

B. As depicted in Figure 13.1, an anesthetic cream is being applied to decrease needlestick pain. (pp. 413–414)

8.

D. After the capillary blood gas collection, pressure should be applied over the puncture site with a dry gauze sponge until the bleeding stops. (p. 424)

9.

D. The venipuncture technique for infants as shown in Figure 13.2 requires the positioning of the needle at a 15-degree angle over the vein. (p. 431)

10.

D. When a skin puncture is performed on an infant or a child, hematology specimens are collected first to minimize platelet clumping. (p. 416)

11.

B. The infant's heel should have a sterile gauze pressed against the skin puncture site after blood collection to avoid the formation of a hematoma. (p. 420)

12.

B. Children who are 3–5 years old perceive pain from a needlestick as a punishment for bad behavior. (p. 411)

13.

A. The total blood volume of a premature infant is calculated by multiplying the weight in kilograms by 115 mL/kg. (p. 416)

14.

B. In the United States, neonatal blood screening for PKU and hypothyroidism is mandatory by law. (p. 424)

15.

D. The age group of 13–17 years old is embarrassed to show fear during venipuncture. (p. 409)

16.

B. When performing skin puncture on infants or children, the phlebotomist collects the hematology specimens first to minimize platelet clumping. (p. 416)

17.

C. If a venipuncture is needed for larger amounts of blood on a child younger than 2 years of age, the medial wrist and the scalp are the two acceptable sites for venipuncture. (p. 428)

18.

D. Newborns are routinely screened through blood analysis for various metabolic and genetic defects that include PKU, congenital hypothyroidism, galactosemia, homocystinuria, congenital adrenal hyperplasia, and sickle cell disease. (pp. 424–425)

19.

B. Compared with skin puncture, venipuncture on a child is needed for the collection of specimens for blood cultures. (pp. 428–429)

20.

C. Some complications that can occur due to neonatal heel sticks include celluitis, osteomyelitis, and scarring of the heel. (p. 416)

21.

B. If 20 mL of blood is collected from a newborn infant (weighing 4.0 kg) over a 2-day period, that is equivalent to approximately 4% of the infant's total blood volume. (p. 416)

22.

A. Figure 13.3 shows the median cubital vein that is usually the best to be used for blood collection in children. (pp. 428, 336)

23.

D. Children with spina bifida are particularly sensitive to latex, and thus a tourniquet that is latex-free should be used when collecting their blood. (p. 415)

24.

A. For pediatric skin puncture, the following equipment is needed. (p. 417):

1. sterile automatic disposable pediatric safety lancet devices
2. 70% isopropyl alcohol swabs in sterile packages
3. sterile cotton balls or gauze sponges
4. plastic capillary collection tubes and sealer
5. microcollection containers and Unopettes
6. glass slides for smears
7. puncture-resistant sharps container
8. disposable gloves (nonlatex if child is allergic)
9. compress (towel or washcloth) to warm heel, if necessary
10. marking pen
11. laboratory request slips or labels

25.

D. A 23-gauge safety winged infusion set (butterfly needle) is used for the scalp vein venipuncture. (p. 431)

26.

B. For blood culture collections from infants, chlorhexidine gluconate swabs should be used rather than iodine for their sensitive skin. (p. 430)

27.

C. The infant's heel should be prewarmed for 3–5 minutes prior to the heel stick. (p. 418)

28.

B. Osteomyelitis can result from multiple deep skin punctures on an infant's heel. (p. 416)

29.

B. When collecting blood from a saline lock on a child, the blood collector must check the patency of the line by flushing the catheter cap with a small amount of normal saline. (p. 433)

30.

B. When performing a heel stick on an infant, position the infant in the supine position (face up). (p. 418)

31.

D. Blood spot testing for neonatal screening is performed before the newborn is 72 hours old. (p. 425)

32.

C. Blood collection for neonatal screening to detect metabolic and genetic defects occurs on the infant's lateral or medial plantar surface of the heel. (p. 426)

33.

C. Figure 13.4 shows blood being collected for neonatal metabolic screening. (p. 426)

34.

C. For psychological reasons, the best location for a painful procedure such as phlebotomy is a treatment room away from the child's bed or playroom. (pp. 411–412)

35.

D. After blood is collected for PKU testing, the card must thoroughly dry in a horizontal position for a minimum of 4 hours. (p. 427)

36.

C. Depression is an emotional factor associated with geriatric patients. (p. 436)

37.

D. An automatic lancet should be used for the finger stick to a child, and the stick should not exceed 2.0 mm for small children. (p. 416)

38.

A. To collect blood from an IV line in a child, a syringe that can enter a needleless cannula is the safe method for blood collection. Thus, after collection, a transfer device is needed to transfer the blood to the vacuum tubes. (pp. 434–435)

39.

D. OSHA mandates that latex or silicone membrane ports be used on CVCs because the ports allow penetration with a needleless access device and can easily be disinfected before entry. (p. 432)

40.

C. When performing venipuncture on a child's arm, it is recommended to use a winged safety infusion needle that is 23-gauge. (p. 429)

41.

C. The preferred site for a heel stick is the medial or lateral aspect of the heel. (pp. 416–417)

42.

C. A 10-mL blood sample taken from a premature or newborn infant is equivalent to 5–10% of the infant's total blood volume. (p. 416)

43.

D. In the United States, neonatal blood screening for phenylketonuria (PKU) and hypothyroidism is mandatory by law. These diseases can result in severe abnormalities, including mental retardation. (p. 424)

44.

C. A premature infant weighing 2.0 kg will have a total blood volume of 115 mL/kg × 2 kg = 230 mL. (p. 416)

45.

B. Blood cultures require large amounts of blood that must be collected by venipuncture. (pp. 428–429)

46.

D. When collecting blood from a child's long-term CVC, use a 10 mL syringe. (pp. 434–435)

47.

B. EMLA is a topical anesthetic applied to the child's arm before venipuncture. (p. 413)

48.

D. For children older than 1 year, the palmar surface of the tip of the third or fourth finger is most frequently used. (p. 428)

49.

D. The topical anesthetic EMLA, which is an emulsion of lidocaine and prilocaine, can be applied to an infant or child to alleviate pain from venipuncture. (p. 413)

50.

A. The angle of the needle for a pediatric venipuncture should be 30 degrees or less with the skin surface. (pp. 337, 428–430)

CHAPTER

14 Point-of-Care Collections

chapter objectives

Upon completion of Chapter 14, the learner is responsible for the following:

1. List two terms that are synonymous with point-of-care testing.
2. Identify four analytes whose levels can be determined through point-of-care testing.
3. Describe the most widely used application of point-of-care testing.
4. Define quality assurance and its requirements in point-of-care testing.
5. Describe the equipment that is used to perform the bleeding-time test.

DIRECTIONS Each of the questions or incomplete statements below is followed by four suggested answers or completions. Select one answer that is best in each case.

1. The bleeding-time test is used to:
   A. check for vascular abnormalities
   B. diagnose diabetes mellitus
   C. determine whether the patient's blood pressure is low
   D. access liver glycogen stores

2. Figure 14.1 shows the skin puncture on the patient's arm in preparation for what analysis/analyses?
   A. capillary blood gases
   B. bleeding-time test
   C. troponin T
   D. Bili*Check*

3. The following materials and/or supplies are needed for the Surgicutt procedure *except*:
   A. blood pressure cuff
   B. butterfly-type bandage
   C. disposable gloves
   D. vacuum blood collection tube with EDTA

4. Results from point-of-care (POC) testing should contain:
   A. the same information as results from a clinical laboratory
   B. the same information as results from a clinical laboratory and a note that the results are from a bedside (or home) rather than from the clinical lab
   C. a signature from the patient
   D. informed consent from the patient

FIGURE 14.1

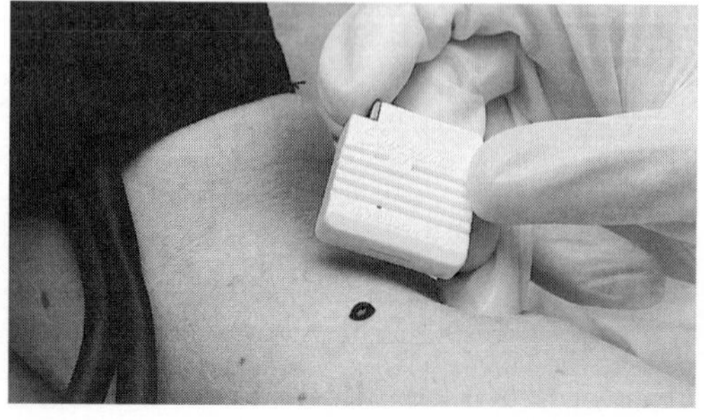

5. If the patient's bleeding time is longer than the normal limits, which of the following laboratory tests may be needed?
   A. alkaline phosphatase level
   B. acid phosphatase level
   C. platelet function screening
   D. BUN result

6. Which of the following POC instruments uses a microcuvette to measure the analyte?
   A. Accu-Chek
   B. FreeStyle
   C. HemoCue
   D. Nova Biomedical Stat Profile pHOx

7. Quality in POC testing requires that glucose control material be based on the use of:
   A. sterile liquid controls
   B. whole blood controls
   C. sterile saline controls
   D. plasma from pooled patients' blood

8. What POC testing procedure is used to test for the maintenance of blood glucose levels?
   A. troponins T or 1
   B. hemoglobin A1c
   C. prothrombin time (PT)
   D. hemoglobin

9. The pancreas produces:
   A. insulin
   B. glucose
   C. cholesterol
   D. hemoglobin

10. What blood collection equipment is *not* required for the testing apparatus shown in Figure 14.2?
    A. gauge sponges
    B. gray-topped evacuated blood collection tube
    C. gloves
    D. 70% isopropyl alcohol swabs

11. What POC test has been determined to be more accurate than the hematocrit test in diagnosis and treatment of anemia?
    A. RBC count
    B. WBC count
    C. hemoglobin
    D. packed cell volume (PCV)

FIGURE 14.2 HemoCue, Inc., Lake Forest, CA.

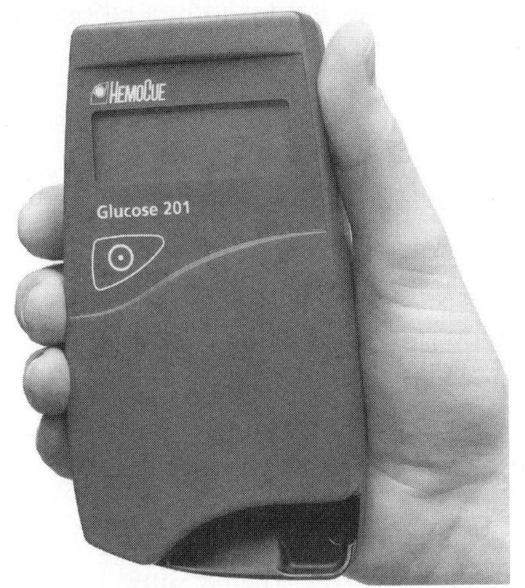

12. What POC testing procedure is used for coagulation testing?
    A. NOVA Biomedical Stat Profile
    B. OraQuick assay
    C. HemoCue
    D. Hemochron Jr.

13. Which POC instrument is used to analyze whether a patient has a heart or lung disorder?
    A. HemoCue beta-glucose analyzer
    B. NOVA Biomedical Stat Profile pHOx analyzer
    C. CoaguChek System
    D. HemoCue beta-hemoglobin analyzer

14. Most rapid methods for glucose testing require:
    A. serum
    B. plasma
    C. skin puncture blood
    D. RBCs

15. Which of the following blood analytes is *not* measured through POC testing?
    A. cholesterol
    B. glucose
    C. troponin T
    D. zinc

16. What is troponin T?
    A. a coagulation factor to decrease bleeding
    B. instrument that is used to test T_4
    C. analyte to detect heart damage
    D. analyte to detect pancreatic damage

17. Which of the following is referred to as the good cholesterol and thus is important to collect blood and test for its value?
    A. LDL cholesterol
    B. total cholesterol
    C. HDL cholesterol
    D. cholinesterase

18. Hemostasis refers to:
    A. steady-state condition
    B. arrest or stopping of bleeding
    C. localized leakage of blood
    D. lack of flow of lymph fluid

19. The Cholestech LDX System can obtain blood levels for which of the following analytes?
    A. C-peptide
    B. troponins
    C. triglycerides
    D. creatine kinase

20. The International Technidyne Corp. (ITC) ProTime Microcoagulation System uses which of the following for testing the analytes?
    A. only capillary blood
    B. only venous blood
    C. venous or arterial blood
    D. capillary or venous blood

21. Which of the following POC analyzers has been designed to use for accurate measurements on neonatal blood?
    A. INRatio Meter
    B. Roche Tropt
    C. Statstrip Glucose Analyzer
    D. Roche CoaguChek System

22. Which of the following is another term for PCV?
    A. anemia
    B. hematocrit
    C. hemoglobin
    D. INRatio

23. Which of the following can be used to measure hemoglobin with the HemoCue beta-hemoglobin analyzer?
    A. only arterial or venous blood
    B. only venous or capillary blood
    C. venous, capillary, or arterial blood
    D. only capillary blood

24. Which of the following procedures helps to reduce potential scarring from the Surgicutt bleeding-time test?
    A. Apply a butterfly-type bandage to the incision site.
    B. Provide a small stitch to the incision site.
    C. Apply gauze and tape to the incision site.
    D. Apply a small piece of moleskin to the incision site.

25. What does ACT refer to in a laboratory testing?
    A. hemoglobin
    B. activated clotting time
    C. bleeding-time test
    D. platelet aggregation

26. Which of the following terms is synonymous with POC testing?
    A. alternate-site testing
    B. protection of collection testing
    C. bleeding-time testing
    D. capillary blood gas testing

FIGURE 14.3

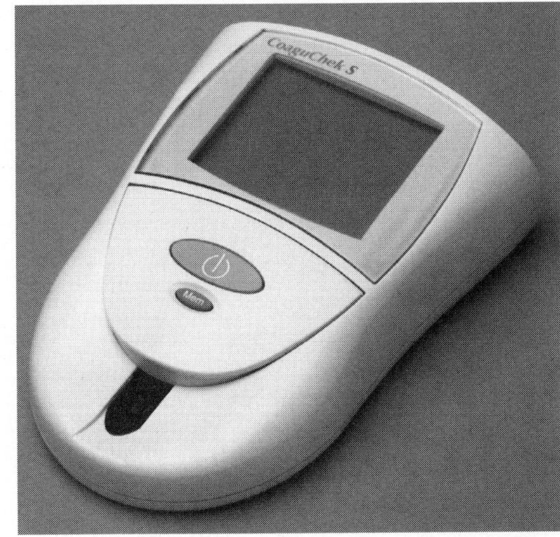

27. The instrument in Figure 14.3 measures:
    A. PCV
    B. PT
    C. RBCs
    D. pCO2

28. For the health care worker who is to perform a glucose POC test, which of the following is *essential* information?
    A. the type of blood that can be used for the POC test—from a fingerstick and/or blood from a venipuncture
    B. the blood type of the patient
    C. the patient age group that the blood instrument can be used for
    D. both A and C are correct

29. Which of the following laboratory tests determines whether the blood is too acidic or too alkaline?
    A. Ca^{++}
    B. pH
    C. TCO_2
    D. PCV

30. A less than normal number of erythrocytes is referred to as:
    A. hemoglobin
    B. anemia
    C. diabetes
    D. arthritis

31. Interpretation of a quality control chart is based on the fact that for a normal distribution:
    A. 99% of the values are within 3 SD of the mean
    B. 99% of the values are within 2 SD of the mean
    C. 95% of the values are within 3 SD of the mean
    D. 95% of the values are within 1 SD of the mean

32. Which of the following is released from the pancreas and has a major effect on blood glucose levels?
    A. ACTH
    B. insulin
    C. thyroxine
    D. renin

33. In POC testing, the purpose of EQC is to:
    A. calibrate the blood glucose standards
    B. test the instrument's internal and analyte circuits
    C. monitor if the blood sample has been hemolyzed
    D. determine if the blood specimen should be analyzed in the clinical laboratory

34. Which of the following abbreviations refer(s) to the term hematocrit?
    A. Hct and crit
    B. CBC
    C. hemo scan
    D. retic

35. Na^+, K^+, Cl^-, and HCO^- are usually referred to as:
    A. electrolytes
    B. blood gases
    C. hormones
    D. coagulation factors

36. In terms of quality control procedures, SD stands for:
    A. short distance
    B. standard deviation
    C. shared diameter
    D. standard dimension

37. Which of the following POC instruments can be used to determine the hematology parameters that include hemoglobin, hematocrit, and platelet aggregation?
    A. Ichor Automated Cell Counter
    B. INRatio Meter
    C. HemoCue beta-hemoglobin analyzer
    D. NOVA Biomedical Stat Profile

38. Which of the following is *not* a POC blood glucose monitor?
    A. NOVA Biomedical Stat Profile pHOx Plus
    B. INRatio Meter
    C. One Touch Ultra
    D. FreeStyle

39. The Roche Tropt POC test uses which of the following for the assay?
    A. capillary blood
    B. capillary or venous blood
    C. venous blood
    D. arterial blood

40. The HemoCue beta-glucose analyzer can obtain test results from:
    A. only capillary or venous blood
    B. only venous or arterial blood

FIGURE 14.4

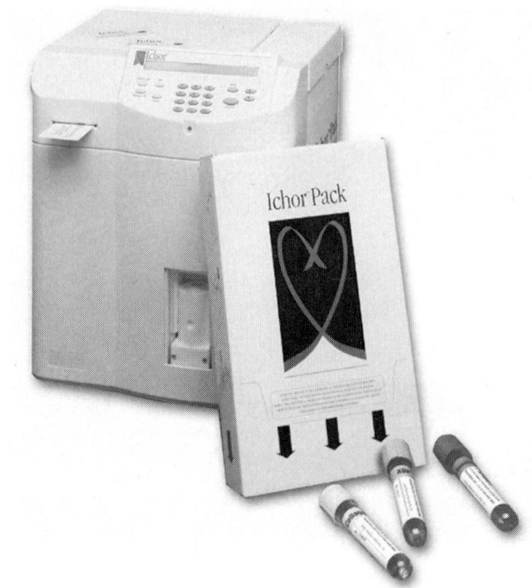

    C. only arterial or capillary blood
    D. arterial, capillary, or venous blood

41. In the development of a quality control record, tolerance limits are determined by pooling the data of laboratory results obtained during what test period?
    A. 5-day test period
    B. 10-day test period
    C. 15-day test period
    D. 30-day test period

42. Figure 14.4 shows an instrument for:
    A. urinalysis
    B. hematology parameters
    C. chemistry parameters
    D. blood gas measurement

43. Figure 14.5 is a POC analyzer used for the measurement of:
    A. urinalysis
    B. hemoglobin
    C. blood coagulation
    D. glucose

FIGURE 14.5

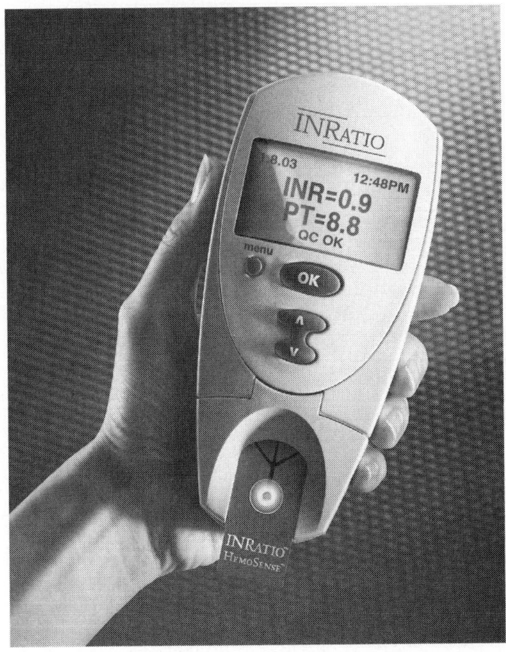

44. Which of the following is used in POC laboratory testing to monitor blood coagulation?
    A. pCO_2 and pH
    B. INR and PT
    C. Hct and Hb
    D. troponin T

45. For the HemoCue beta-glucose testing procedure:
    A. the dorsal vein is the best location for the blood collection
    B. the first three drops of blood should be wiped away after the incision
    C. apply a latex-free tourniquet for the procedure
    D. use a safety syringe so that the elderly person's arm will not be damaged from vacuum tubes

46. Using Figure 14.6, which of the following statements is true?
    A. On day 7, the glucose control was out of the 2 SD control range.
    B. On day 8, the glucose control was the same as the patient's value.
    C. On day 3, the glucose control had a mean value of 100 mg/dL.
    D. On day 1, the glucose control was too low.

47. Using Figure 14.6 as shown also in Question 46, identify the tolerance limits for the glucose control.
    A. 91–100 mg/dL
    B. 100–109 mg/dL
    C. 91–109 mg/dL
    D. 96–105 mg/dL

48. When referring to a quality control chart such as the one in Figure 14.6, what do the comments indicate?
    A. There was a problem on days 2 and 5.
    B. There was a dead battery on day 5.
    C. Preventative maintenance was properly documented.
    D. There was a major problem with the control value on day 3.

49. Which of the following are blood electrolytes that are usually measured by POC?
    A. pH, pO_2, and pCO_2
    B. sodium, potassium, chloride
    C. PT and INR
    D. troponin T, TCO_2

50. Which of the following blood assays can assist in the diagnosis and evaluation of anemia?
    A. Na^+ and K^+
    B. hemoglobin and hematocrit
    C. glucose and insulin
    D. pH and pCO_2

FIGURE 14.6

Glucose Monitor

QUALITY CONTROL RECORD

PRACTICE NAME: Med Mobile Clinic

INSTRUMENT: Glucose Monitor - Mobile Clinic

CONTROL LOT#: 54539 EXPIRATION DATE: 03/05/12

DIRECTOR SIGNATURE/DATE:

NAME/LEVEL: Accu Glucose/Normal

TEST Glucose *Glucose Monitor UNITS: mg/dl

LOWER LIMIT: 91 MEAN: 100 UPPER LIMIT: 109

DATE	NO.	VALUE	TECH	COMMENT	DATE	NO.	VALUE	TECH	COMMENT
2/8/08	1	99	KBM			17			
2/9/08	2	103	KBM	prev. maintenance		18			
2/10/08	3	100	KBM			19			
2/11/08	4	100	KBM			20			
2/12/08	5	105	KBM			21			
2/15/08	6	97	KBM			22			
2/16/08	7	95	KBM			23			
2/17/08	8	96	KBM	new battery		24			
2/18/08	9	103	KBM			25			
2/19/08	10	100	KBM			26			
2/20/08	11	103	KBM			27			
2/21/08	12	97	KBM			28			
	13					29			
	14					30			
	15					31			
	16								

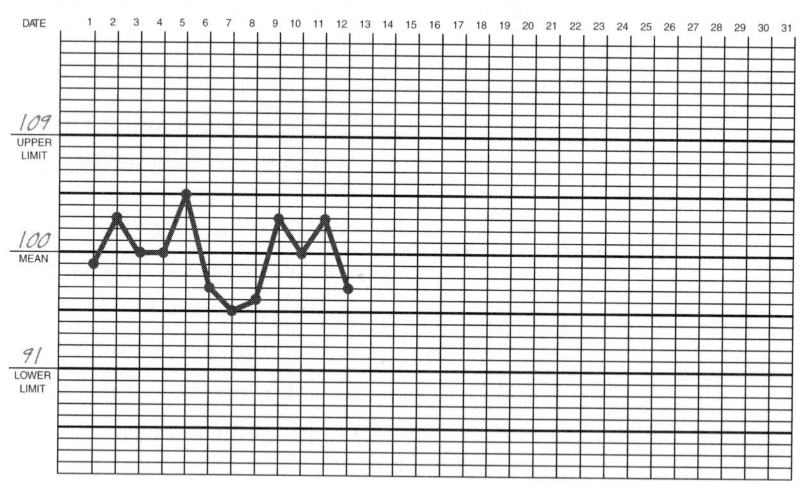

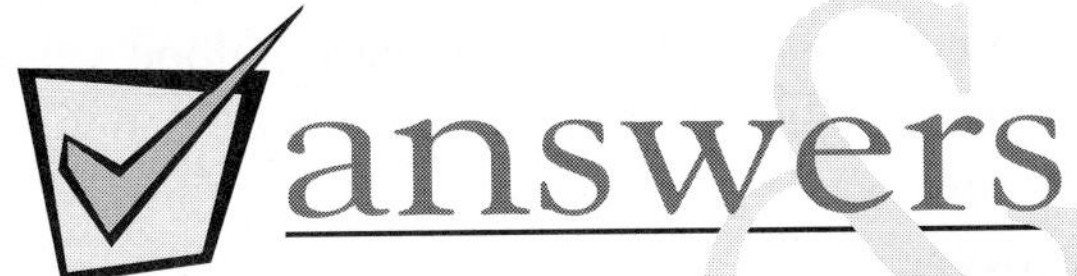

answers & rationales

1.

A. The bleeding-time test is used to check for vascular abnormalities. This diagnostic test has been used as a test for hemostasis (i.e., the stoppage of bleeding by the body). (p. 456)

2.

B. Figure 14.1 shows the skin puncture on the patient's arm in preparation for the bleeding-time test. The procedure is performed on the forearm of the patient and by recording the length of time required for bleeding to cease. (pp. 458–459)

3.

D. The blood pressure cuff, butterfly-type bandage, and disposable gloves are needed for the Surgicutt procedure. This procedure does not use vacuum blood collection tubes. (p. 457).

4.

B. Results from POC testing should contain the same information as results from a clinical laboratory plus a note that the results are from a bedside (or home) rather than from the clinical laboratory. (p. 450)

5.

C. If the patient's bleeding time is longer than the normal limits, platelet function screening assays might be needed. (p. 456)

6.

C. Both the HemoCue beta-glucose analyzer and the HemoCue beta-hemoglobin system use a microcuvette to measure the analyte. (p. 447)

7.

B. Quality in POC testing requires that glucose control material be based on the use of whole blood controls similar to the patient's specimen in order to determine if the analytic system is working properly. (p. 450)

8.

B. Hemoglobin A1c is a procedure to test for the maintenance of blood glucose levels. (p. 460)

9.

A. Insulin is a chemical that is released into the bloodstream by the pancreas when glucose levels in the blood increase. (p. 446)

10.

B. The HemoCue glucose meter shown in Figure 14.2 uses blood from skin puncture, venipuncture, or a flushed heparin line. Thus, gauge sponges, gloves, and 70% isopropyl alcohol swabs are needed, but a gray-topped evacuated blood collection tube is not needed for the glucose analysis performed on this POC instrument. (pp. 448–449)

11.

C. The hemoglobin test has been determined by the American Medical Association (AMA) to be more accurate than the hematocrit test in diagnosis and treatment of anemia. (p. 455)

12.

D. The Hemochron Jr. point-of-care testing instrument is used for coagulation testing. (p. 454)

13.

B. The NOVA Biomedical Stat Profile pHOx analyzer measures blood gases (pH, pCO_2, pO_2) that can detect whether a patient has a heart or lung disorder. (p. 452)

14.

C. Most rapid methods for glucose testing require skin puncture blood. (p. 445)

15.

D. Cholesterol, glucose, and troponin T can all be measured through POC testing. Zinc is a trace element that requires special collection in a trace element (royal blue) vacuum collection tube and special testing procedures. (pp. 446–447, 453, 456)

16.

C. Troponin T is measured by POC instruments to detect heart damage. (p. 453)

17.

C. HDL cholesterol is referred to as the good cholesterol since increased blood values protect the patient from heart disease. (p. 456)

18.

B. Hemostasis refers to the arrest or stopping of bleeding. (p. 457)

19.

C. The Cholestech LDX System can obtain blood levels for triglycerides. (p. 456)

20.

D. The ITC ProTime Microcoagulation System uses capillary or venous blood that is collected into the disposable cuvette for insertion into the instrument for measurement. (p. 454)

21.

C. Statstrip Glucose analyzer has been designed to use for accurate measurements of glucose on neonatal blood. (p. 447)

22.

B. PCV stands for packed cell volume and is another term for hematocrit that represents the volume of circulating blood that is occupied by RBCs. (p. 455)

23.

C. Venous, capillary, or arterial blood can be used to measure hemoglobin with the HemoCue beta-hemoglobin analyzer. (p. 455)

24.

A. Applying a nonallergenic butterfly-type bandage for 24 hours helps to reduce potential scarring from the Surgicutt bleeding-time test. (p. 457)

25.

B. ACT stands for activated clotting time. (p. 454)

26.

A. The demand for POC testing is increasing because rapid turnaround of laboratory results is necessary for prompt medical decision making. This type of testing occurs at or near the point of direct contact with the patient. Therefore, the terms used for these direct laboratory services include decentralized lab testing, on-site testing, alternate-site testing, near-patient testing, patient-focused testing, and bedside testing. (p. 445)

27.

B. Figure 14.3 is the CoaguChek System that measures PT. (p. 453)

28.

D. For the health care worker who is to perform a glucose POC test, he or she needs to know what type of blood—blood from a finger stick and/or that from venipuncture—can be used to perform glucose determination with the POC instrument and the patient age group that the blood instrument can be used for. (pp. 446–447)

29.

B. The blood pH determines whether the blood is too acidic or too alkaline. (p. 452)

30.

B. A state of less than normal number of erythrocytes is referred to as anemia. (p. 455)

31.

A. Interpretation of a quality control chart is based on the fact that for a normal distribution, 99% of the values are within 3 SD of the mean. (p. 450)

32.

B. Insulin is released from the pancreas and has a major effect on blood glucose levels. Normally, insulin is released into the bloodstream after meals when glucose levels increase; it causes glucose to be absorbed from the blood into the body tissues where it is used for energy. In patients with diabetes mellitus, glucose is not properly absorbed by the tissues, and the glucose levels within the blood increase. If a patient has an elevated level, he or she can enter a state of metabolic acidosis, which in turn may result in shock and death. (p. 446)

33.

B. In point-of-care testing, the purpose of "electronic quality control" (EQC) is to test the instrument's internal and analyte circuits. (p. 450)

34.

A. The abbreviations Hct and crit are synonymous with the term "hematocrit." (p. 455)

35.

A. Na^+, K^+, Cl^-, and HCO^- are usually referred to as electrolytes. (p. 453)

36.

B. SD stands for standard deviation. It is used in quality control procedures to determine variation from the mean, or the average value that is expected. In a normal distribution of values, 95% of the time the values will be within 2 standard deviations of the mean, and 99% of the values are within 3 standard deviations of the mean. (p. 450)

37.

A. Ichor Automated Cell Counter can be used to determine the hematology parameters that include hemoglobin, hematocrit, and platelet aggregation. (pp. 455–456)

38.

B. The INRatio Meter is used for blood coagulation monitoring, not for glucose testing. (pp. 453–454)

39.

C. The Roche Tropt POC test uses venous blood (heparin or EDTA) for the troponin T assay. (p. 453)

40.

D. The HemoCue beta-glucose analyzer can obtain test results from arterial, capillary, or venous blood. (p. 448)

41.

D. In the development of a quality control record, tolerance limits are determined by pooling the data of laboratory results obtained during a 20 to 30 day test period. (p. 450)

42.

B. Figure 14.4 shows the Ichor automated cell counter (Helena Laboratories, Beaumont, TX), an instrument used for hematology analysis in acute adult and pediatric patient management. (p. 455)

43.

C. Figure 14.5 is a POC analyzer used for the measurement of blood coagulation. (p. 454)

44.

B. INR (International Normalized Ratio) and PT (prothrombin time) are used in POC laboratory testing to monitor blood coagulation. (p. 453)

45.

B. The HemoCue beta-glucose testing procedure requires that the first three drops of blood be wiped away after a skin puncture. (p. 448)

46.

C. As shown in Figure 14.6, on day 3, the glucose control had a mean value of 100 mg/dL. This is normal and expected. (p. 451)

47.

C. As shown in Figure 14.6, the tolerance limit range for the glucose control is from 91 mg/dL (lower limit) to 109 mg/dL (upper limit). (pp. 450–451)

48.

C. As shown in Figure 14.6, the comments indicate that preventative maintenance was properly documented, and a battery was replaced, as is probably indicated in the required maintenance of the instrument. (p. 451)

49.

B. Sodium, potassium, and chloride are blood electrolytes usually measured by POC. (p. 453)

50.

B. Laboratory evaluations of hemoglobin and hematocrit assist in the diagnosis and evaluation of anemia. (p. 455)

CHAPTER

15 Arterial, Intravenous (IV), and Special Collection Procedures

chapter objectives

Upon completion of Chapter 15, the learner is responsible for the following:

1. List the steps and equipment in blood culture collections.
2. Discuss the requirements for the glucose and lactose tolerance tests.
3. Explain the special precautions and types of equipment needed to collect arterial blood gases.
4. Differentiate cannulas from fistulas.
5. List the special requirements for collecting blood through intravenous (IV) catheters.
6. Differentiate therapeutic phlebotomy from autologous transfusion.
7. Describe the special precautions needed to collect blood in therapeutic drug monitoring (TDM) procedures.
8. List the types of patient specimens that are needed for trace metal analyses.

DIRECTIONS Each of the questions or incomplete statements below is followed by four suggested answers or completions. Select one answer that is best in each case.

1. Which of the following should occur first in the collection protocol during the collection of blood for blood cultures by the butterfly assembly procedure?
   A. Insert the butterfly needle into the venipuncture site.
   B. Transfer the blood to the aerobic bottle.
   C. Transfer the blood to the anaerobic bottle.
   D. Disinfect the rubber septum on the blood culture bottles with 70% isopropyl alcohol.

2. Which of the following can lead to deferral of a person from blood donation? The potential donor has:
   A. purulent skin lesions on his or her arms
   B. a poison ivy rash on his or her arms
   C. psoriasis skin lesions on his or her arms
   D. acne skin lesions on his or her arms

3. Which of the following sites is *not* recommended to collect ABGs?
   A. ulnar artery
   B. radial artery
   C. femoral artery
   D. brachial artery

4. What anesthetic should be used for the collection of a specimen for ABG analysis?
   A. heparin
   B. EDTA
   C. lidocaine
   D. sodium citrate

5. An artificial shunt in which the vein and artery have been fused through surgery is usually found in:
   A. cardiac patients
   B. renal dialysis patients
   C. patients with liver disease
   D. patients with leg amputations

6. Therapeutic phlebotomy is used in the treatment of:
   A. megaloblastic anemia
   B. hereditary hemochromatosis
   C. chronic anemia
   D. iron-deficiency anemia

7. Blood glucose levels are measured for patients undergoing:
   A. Allen test
   B. blood gas analysis
   C. lactose tolerance test
   D. therapeutic phlebotomy

8. Which of the following drugs has a shorter half-life and therefore requires exact timing in blood collection for its therapeutic level?
   A. tobramycin
   B. phenobarbital
   C. digoxin
   D. digitoxin

9. Which of the following evacuated tubes is preferred for the collection of ABG analysis?
   A. yellow-topped evacuated tube
   B. green-topped evacuated tube

C. light-blue-topped evacuated tube
D. no evacuated tube

10. During a GTT, which procedure is acceptable?
    A. A standard amount of glucose drink is given to the patient; then a fasting blood collection is performed.
    B. The patient should be encouraged to drink water throughout the procedure.
    C. The patient is allowed to chew sugarless gum after the first blood specimen is collected.
    D. All the patient's specimens are timed from the fasting collection.

11. Normally, after an adult patient ingests the 75 or 100 g of glucose in the GTT, the glucose level should return to normal within how many minutes?
    A. 30
    B. 60
    C. 120
    D. 180

12. Which of the following is used frequently for collection of blood specimens for the genetic molecular tests?
    A. green-topped evacuated collection tube
    B. lavender-topped evacuated collection tube
    C. royal-blue-topped evacuated collection tube
    D. pink-topped evacuated collection tube

13. As shown in Figure 15.1, the performance of this test:
    A. determines collateral circulation of the radial and femoral arteries
    B. checks for venous abnormalities
    C. shows a positive result if the hand fills with blood within 5–10 seconds
    D. provides a quick method to assess the brachial artery's pressure

14. Which of the following tubes must be collected first?
    A. yellow-topped evacuated tube
    B. red-topped evacuated tube
    C. light-blue-topped evacuated tube
    D. royal-blue-topped evacuated tube

15. To help minimize the incidence of dizziness, fainting, or other reactions to blood loss, blood donors are encouraged to eat within how many hours of donating blood?
    A. 9
    B. 8
    C. 7
    D. 6

FIGURE 15.1

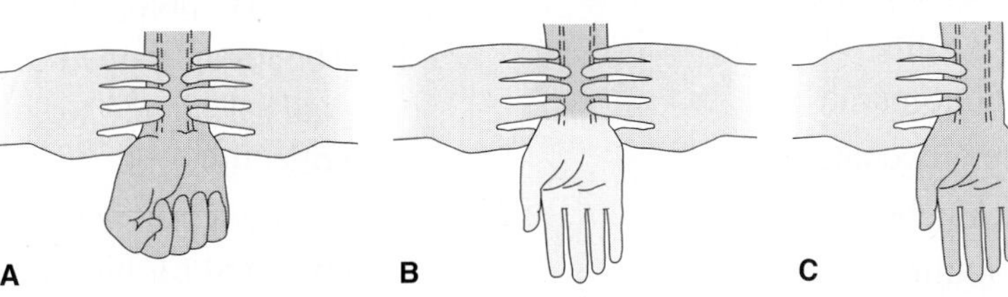

16. An autologous transfusion is used to prevent which of the following possibilities?
    A. Polycythemia will develop in the transfused patient.
    B. Antigens will form in the transfused patient.
    C. Antibodies will form in the transfused patient.
    D. The transfused patient will develop diabetes mellitus.

17. Which of the following is not mandatory information to be collected on a potential blood donor?
    A. gender
    B. race
    C. birth date
    D. reason for deferrals

18. Which of the following guidelines must the patient abide by to properly prepare himself or herself for the GTT?
    A. The patient's carbohydrate intake must not exceed 20 g per day for 3 days before the GTT.
    B. The patient must not eat anything for 12 hours before the GTT but should not fast for more than 14 hours before the test.
    C. The patient should take corticosteroids 2 days before the GTT.
    D. The patient should vigorously exercise within 8–12 hours before the GTT.

19. If a patient is sensitive or allergic to iodine, then in venipuncture site preparation for the blood culture collection, the phlebotomist should use which of the following?
    A. 1% PVP without iodine
    B. chlorhexidine gluconate
    C. soap/acetone alcohol
    D. 0.75% PVP–iodine

20. Which of the following items is *not* usually kept on file for every blood donor indefinitely?
    A. age
    B. a written consent form signed by the donor
    C. a record of reason for deferrals
    D. a written consent form signed by the donor's parent

21. Which of the following procedures requires blood collection for trough- and peak-level determinations?
    A. blood culture collections
    B. modified Allen test
    C. blood collection through CVCs
    D. TDM

22. For CVC blood collections, which of the following blood analytes has to have 8–10 mL of blood discarded from the line before another separate syringe is used to collect an additional amount for the analyte test?
    A. PT
    B. LD
    C. ALT
    D. AST

23. Which of the following is a true statement regarding blood culture blood collections?
    A. Microbiology culture bottles with the vacuum can be used for direct draw through the needle holder evacuated tube system if the top of the bottles are properly prepped.
    B. The green-topped evacuated tube is especially designed for blood culture collections.
    C. If only 3 mL or less of blood can be collected for blood cultures, place the

entire amount of blood in the aerobic bottle.

D. Povidone is superior over iodine tincture in combating the contamination of blood collection sites for blood cultures.

24. Figure 15.2 shows swabbing of the arm in concentric circles in preparation of collecting blood for:
    A. TDM
    B. toxicology studies
    C. blood cultures
    D. lactose tolerance test

25. For a donor to donate blood, his or her oral temperature must not exceed:
    A. 35°C
    B. 37.5°C
    C. 38.7°C
    D. 39.5°F

26. The term "homologous transfusion" refers to:
    A. a patient who donates his or her own blood before anticipated surgery
    B. involving one individual as both donor and recipient
    C. blood that can be transfused from a donor who had therapeutic bleeding
    D. the stoppage of the circulation of blood in a part of the body as the blood is transfused

FIGURE 15.2

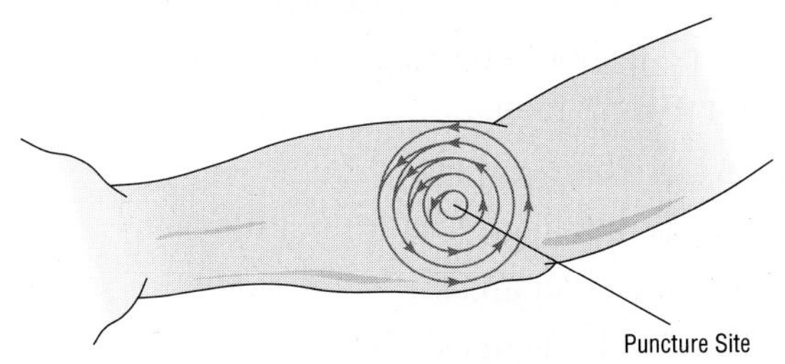

27. A false-negative blood culture is more likely to occur if:
    A. the anaerobic blood culture bottle is inoculated with blood and air
    B. the indwelling catheter is used to obtain the culture specimen
    C. too much blood is used for the culture
    D. the health care worker palpates the venipuncture site after it has been prepared without first cleaning the gloved finger

28. Which of the following procedures is frequently used to determine if a patient has septicemia?
    A. GTT
    B. bleeding-time test
    C. blood culture
    D. lactose tolerance test

29. Resin beads to neutralize antibiotics in the blood specimen are used in the:
    A. heparin lock system for IV blood collections
    B. bleeding-time test
    C. blood culture collections
    D. special ABG collections

30. What is the rationale for performing the Allen test?
    A. to test for the possibility of edema
    B. to determine whether the patient's blood pressure is elevated
    C. to determine that the radial and ulnar arteries are providing collateral circulation
    D. to determine whether the oxygen concentration in the radial artery is sufficient for blood collection

31. What is a cannula?
    A. a good source of arterial blood
    B. the fusion of a vein and an artery
    C. a tubular instrument used to gain access to venous blood
    D. an artificial shunt that provides access to arterial blood

32. Before a blood donation, the phlebotomist must always check the blood donor's:
    A. blood glucose value
    B. hematocrit or hemoglobin value
    C. urine glucose value
    D. WBC count

33. *Postprandial* refers to:
    A. 2-hour fasting
    B. 12-hour fasting
    C. after eating
    D. before eating

34. Which of the following evacuated tubes is preferred for the collection of a blood culture specimen?
    A. green-topped evacuated tube
    B. yellow-topped evacuated tube
    C. speckled-topped evacuated tube
    D. light-blue-topped evacuated tube

35. Which of the following can lead to deferral of a person from blood donation?
    A. weighs 110 pounds
    B. has an oral temperature of 37°C
    C. has a hematocrit value of 36%
    D. has a pulse rate of 70 beats per minute

36. Cleansing the venipuncture site before collection of blood culture specimens usually involves the use of:
    A. isopropyl alcohol and peroxide
    B. ethyl alcohol and peroxide
    C. iodine and peroxide
    D. iodine and alcohol

37. Approximately how much blood should be collected for the radial ABG procedure?
    A. 10 mL
    B. 7 mL
    C. 5 mL
    D. 1 mL

38. The health care worker's thumb should not be used for palpating arteries in the arterial puncture procedure because the thumb:
    A. is usually dirty
    B. has less sensitivity than the other fingers
    C. has a pulse that may be confused with the patient's pulse
    D. has more neurons for touching, which interfere in the process of finding the patient's pulse

39. A tubular instrument that is used in kidney patients to gain access to venous blood for dialysis or blood collection is referred to as a:
    A. CVC
    B. cannula
    C. fistula
    D. venous isolator

40. When blood is collected from the radial artery for an ABG collection, the needle should be inserted at an angle of no less than:
    A. 5–10 degrees
    B. 15–20 degrees
    C. 25–30 degrees
    D. 30–45 degrees

41. Which of the following is used to help in the diagnosis of diabetes mellitus?
    A. ABG analysis
    B. PT
    C. TDM
    D. GTT

42. Which of the following tests requires numerous blood collections?
    A. ABG analysis
    B. GTT
    C. bleeding-time test
    D. drug screening

43. Blood gas analyses include testing for:
    A. pH, pH_2O, and pCO_2
    B. pH, pO_2, and pCO_2
    C. pH_2O, pCO_2, and pO_2
    D. pH_2O, pH, and pO_2

44. For the brief physical examination that is required to determine whether a blood donor is generally in good health, the donor's systolic blood pressure should measure no higher than:
    A. 100 mm Hg
    B. 110 mm Hg
    C. 180 mm Hg
    D. 190 mm Hg

45. Which of the following requires two 10-mL disposable syringes with needleless cannula and two 10-mL disposable Luer-Lok syringes filled with sterile normal saline?
    A. blood donation
    B. blood collection through CVCs
    C. blood collection from a blood donor
    D. skin test for allergies

46. Which of the following is the preferred site for blood collection for ABG analysis?
    A. ulnar artery
    B. femoral artery
    C. radial artery
    D. subclavian artery

47. Which of the following is a milk sugar that sometimes cannot be digested by healthy individuals?
    A. glucose
    B. glucagon
    C. lactose
    D. lactate

48. Which of the following is the specimen of choice for testing the pH, pO_2, and pCO_2 of the blood?
    A. arterial blood
    B. venous blood
    C. heparinized plasma
    D. skin puncture blood

49. To obtain the blood trough level for a medication, the patient's blood should be collected:
    A. immediately after the administration of the medication
    B. immediately before the administration of the medication
    C. 2 hours before the administration of the medication
    D. 2 hours after the administration of the medication

50. Which of the following supplies is *not* needed during an arterial puncture for an ABG determination?
    A. gloves
    B. lidocaine
    C. syringe
    D. tourniquet

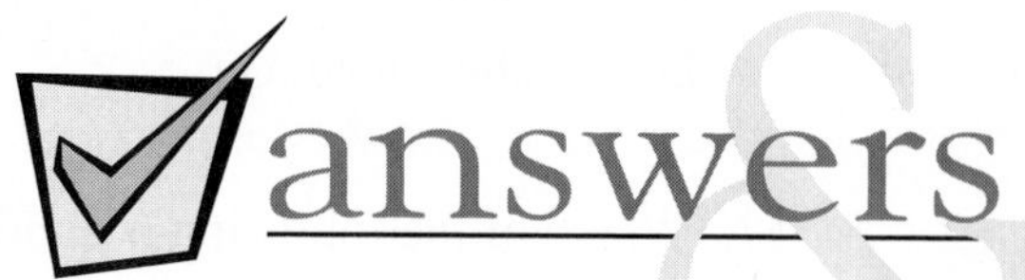

answers & rationales

1.

D. During the collection of blood for blood cultures by the butterfly assembly procedure, the procedural step to disinfect the rubber septum on the blood culture bottles with 70% isopropyl alcohol occurs before insertion of the butterfly needle into the venipuncture site and transfer of blood to the blood culture bottles. (p. 471)

2.

A. Donors with purulent skin lesions, wounds, or severe skin infections should be deferred. The presence of mild skin disorders, such as psoriasis, acne, or a poison ivy rash, does not prohibit an individual from donating blood unless the lesions are in the antecubital area. (p. 493)

3.

A. The ulnar artery is a site that is *not* recommended to collect arterial blood gases. (pp. 479–480)

4.

C. Lidocaine is the anesthetic that should be used to prepare the patient for the collection of an arterial blood gas specimen. (pp. 482–484)

5.

B. A fistula is an artificial shunt in which the vein and artery have been fused through surgery and is a permanent connection tube located in the arm of patients undergoing kidney dialysis. (p. 492)

6.

B. Therapeutic phlebotomy is the intentional removal of blood in conditions in which there is an excessive production of blood cells, as in hereditary hemochromatosis. (p. 494)

7.

C. To determine whether a patient suffers from lactose intolerance, a physician may order a lactose tolerance test, which involves measuring glucose levels over a 2-hour period. (p. 479)

8.

A. The time of collection is much more critical for drugs with shorter half-lives (e.g., gentamicin, tobramycin, and procainamide) than those with longer half-lives (i.e., phenobarbital, digoxin, and digitoxin). (p. 486)

9.

D. For the radial artery blood gas collection, a safety syringe is used, since little or no suction is needed because the blood pulsates and flows quickly into the syringe under its own pressure. (p. 482)

10.

B. During the glucose tolerance test (GTT), the patient is required to have numerous urine collections to test for glucose. Therefore, it is imperative for the patient to drink water during the GTT. However, other liquids have to be avoided, since they will interfere in the test results. (p. 475)

11.

C. Normally, after an adult patient ingests the 75 or 100 g of glucose in the glucose tolerance test (GTT), the glucose level should return to normal within 2 hours. (p. 475)

12.

B. The lavender-topped evacuated collection tube is frequently used for collection of blood specimens for the genetic molecular testing. (p. 487)

13.

C. As shown in Figure 15.1, the performance of this test shows a positive result if the hand fills with blood within 5–10 seconds. (p. 483)

14.

A. If blood culture collections are ordered with other laboratory tests, blood culture specimens (i.e., collected in the SPS yellow-topped evacuated tube) must be collected first to avoid contamination of the blood specimen. (p. 473)

15.

D. To help minimize the incidence of dizziness, fainting, or other reactions to blood loss, blood donors are encouraged to eat within 4–6 hours of donating blood. (p. 493)

16.

C. The autologous transfusion prevents transfusion-transmitted infectious diseases (e.g., hepatitis C) and eliminates the formation of antibodies in the transfused patient. (p. 494)

17.

B. Race is not mandatory information for a potential blood donor, but this information can be useful in screening patients for a specific phenotype. (p. 493)

18.

B. The patient needs to follow these guidelines to prepare for the GTT: (1) the patient's carbohydrate intake must be at least 150 grams per day for 3 days before the GTT, (2) the patient should not eat anything for 12 hours before the GTT, (3) the patient should avoid all possible medications, including corticosteroids, because they will interfere in the GTT, and (4) the patient should avoid exercise for 12 hours before the GTT. (pp. 475–476)

19.

B. If a patient is sensitive or allergic to iodine, use chlorhexidine gluconate to scrub the site of the venipuncture for the blood culture collection. (p. 469)

20.

D. Several items must be kept on file for every donor indefinitely, including age, name, date of birth, a written consent form signed by the donor, and a record of reason for deferrals. The donor, not the donor's parents, consents to his or her own blood collection. (pp. 492–493)

21.

D. So physicians can adequately evaluate the appropriate dosage levels of many drugs, the collection and evaluation of specimens for trough and peak levels are necessary in TDM. (pp. 485–486)

22.

A. It is required to have 8–10 mL of blood aspirated from the CVC line if coagulation studies (e.g., PT, PTT) have been ordered. (p. 490)

23.

C. If only 3 mL or less of blood can be collected for blood cultures, place the entire amount of blood in the aerobic bottle. (p. 472)

24.

C. Figure 15.2 shows swabbing of the arm in concentric circles in preparation of collecting blood for blood cultures. (p. 467)

25.

B. The donor's oral temperature must not exceed 37.5ºC (99.5ºF). (p. 493)

26.

C. The term "homologous transfusion" refers to blood that can be transfused from a donor who had therapeutic bleeding. (p. 495)

27.

A. A false-negative blood culture is more likely to occur if the anaerobic blood culture bottle is inoculated with blood and air. (p. 466)

28.

C. Blood cultures are frequently used to determine if a patient has septicemia (presence of pathogens in the circulating bloodstream, sometimes called blood poisoning). (p. 466)

29.

C. Resin beads that neutralize antibiotics in the patient's blood specimen are used in the blood culture collections. (p. 466)

30.

C. To use the radial artery for blood collection for arterial blood gas analysis, the health care provider must first perform the Allen test to make certain that the ulnar and radial arteries are providing collateral circulation. (p. 483)

31.

C. A cannula is a tubular instrument that is used in patients with kidney disease to gain access to venous blood for dialysis or blood collections. (p. 492)

32.

B. The blood bank phlebotomist must check the blood donor's hematocrit or hemoglobin value before a blood donation, and it must be no less than 12.5 g/dL. (p. 493)

33.

C. *Postprandial* means "after eating." (p. 478)

34.

B. Blood culture specimens need to be collected in SPS (yellow-topped) evacuated tubes. (p. 473)

35.

C. The hematocrit value must be no less than 38% for blood donors. (p. 493)

36.

D. Cleansing the venipuncture site before collection of blood culture specimens usually involves the use of iodine and alcohol. (p. 467)

37.

D. Approximately 1 mL of blood should be collected for the radial ABG procedure. (p. 484)

38.

C. The health care provider's thumb should not be used for palpating arteries in the arterial puncture procedure because the thumb has a pulse that may be confused with the patient's pulse. (p. 483)

39.

B. A cannula is a tubular instrument that is used in kidney patients to gain access to venous blood for dialysis or blood collection. (p. 492)

40.

D. The health care worker should pierce the pulsating artery at a high angle, usually no less than 30–45 degrees against the bloodstream. (p. 484)

41.

D. The glucose tolerance test (GTT) is used to help in the diagnosis of diabetes mellitus. (p. 475)

42.

B. The glucose tolerance test (GTT) is performed by obtaining fasting blood and urine specimens, giving the fasting patient a standard load of glucose, and obtaining subsequent blood and urine specimens at intervals, usually during a 2- or 3-hour period. (pp. 477–478)

43.

B. Blood gas analyses include testing for pH, pO_2, and pCO_2. These tests provide useful information about the respiratory status and the acid-base balance in patients with pulmonary disease or other disorders. (pp. 421, 479)

44.

C. For the brief physical examination required to determine whether a blood donor is in good health, the donor's systolic blood pressure should measure no higher than 180 mm Hg. People with systolic blood pressures out of this range should be deferred as donors. (p. 493)

45.

B. Two 10-mL disposable syringes with needleless cannula and two 10-mL disposable Luer-Lok syringes filled with sterile normal saline are needed for collecting blood through a CVC. (p. 489)

46.

C. When an arterial blood gas analysis is ordered, the health care worker should palpate the radial artery in the radial sulcus of the forearm, since the radial artery in the patient's nondominant hand is usually the best choice. (pp. 482–483)

47.

C. Some otherwise healthy individuals experience difficulty in digesting lactose, a milk sugar. They appear to lack a mucosal lactase enzyme that breaks down the lactose into the simple sugars glucose and galactose. (p. 479)

48.

A. Arterial blood is the specimen of choice for testing the pH, pO_2, and pCO_2 of the blood. Arterial blood is used rather than venous blood because arterial blood has the same composition throughout the body tissues, whereas venous blood has various compositions relative to metabolic activities in body tissues. (pp. 421, 479)

49.

B. To obtain the blood trough level for a medication, the patient's blood should be collected immediately before the administration of the medication. The trough level is the lowest concentration in the patient's serum. (pp. 485–486)

50.

D. No tourniquet is required because the artery has its own strong blood pressure. (pp. 482–484)

CHAPTER

16 Urinalysis, Body Fluids, and Other Specimens

chapter objectives

Upon completion of Chapter 16, the learner is responsible for the following:

1. Identify body fluid specimens, other than blood, that are analyzed in the clinical laboratory, and identify the correct procedures for collecting and/or transporting these specimens to the laboratory.
2. Describe the correct methodology for labeling urine specimens.
3. Identify specimens collected for microbiological, throat, sputum, and nasopharyngeal cultures and the protocol that must be followed when transporting these specimens.
4. List the types of patient specimens that are needed for gastric and sweat chloride analyses.
5. List three types of urine specimen collections and differentiate the uses of the urine specimens obtained from these collections.
6. Instruct a patient on the correct procedure for collecting a timed urine specimen and a midstream clean-catch specimen.

DIRECTIONS Each of the questions or incomplete statements below is followed by four suggested answers or completions. Select one answer that is best in each case.

1. Urine is most concentrated:
   A. in the afternoon
   B. in the evening
   C. after dinner
   D. in the morning

2. Which of the following is collected through a lumbar puncture?
   A. CSF
   B. peritoneal fluid
   C. seminal fluid
   D. pleural fluid

3. As shown in Figure 16.1 which of the following can be measured using the procedure illustrated in the figure?
   A. creatinine clearance
   B. protein
   C. hormones
   D. GTT

FIGURE 16.1

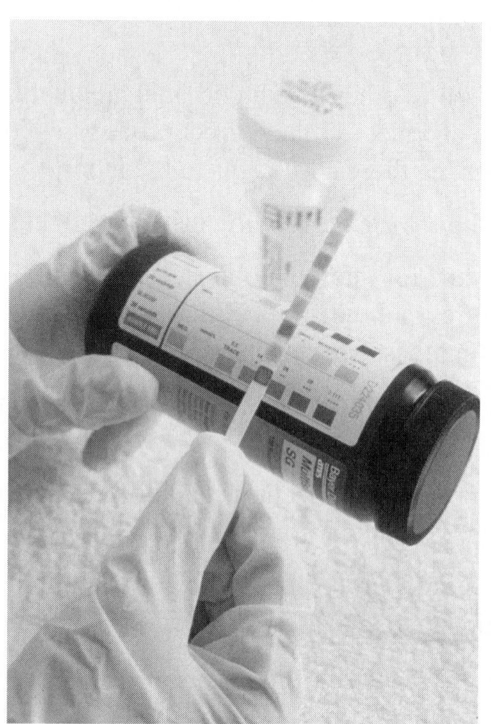

4. As shown in Figure 16.2, the patient is undergoing a:
   A. nasopharyngeal culture collection
   B. gastric analysis
   C. sputum collection
   D. sweat chloride test

5. The *Helicobacter pylori* test is:
   A. gastric analysis
   B. breath analysis
   C. the sweat chloride test
   D. the ColoScreen-ES test

FIGURE 16.2

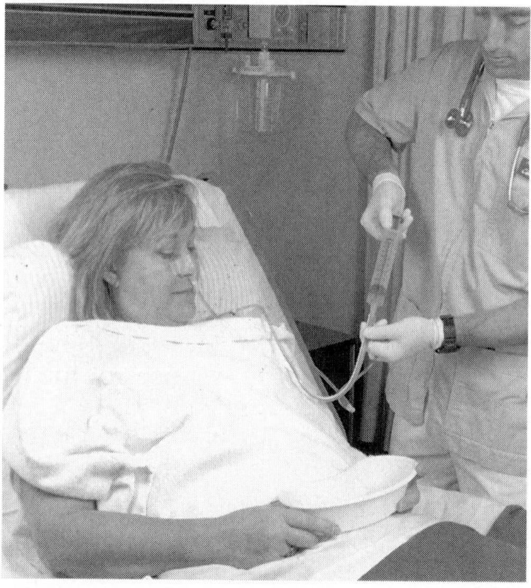

6. Glucose-level determinations for diabetes mellitus testing should occur on what type of urine specimen collection?
   A. fasting specimen
   B. random specimen
   C. clean-catch specimen
   D. first urine of the morning specimen

7. For the TB skin test, the tuberculin syringe should be held at what angle for administration of the antigen?
   A. 5 degrees
   B. 15 degrees
   C. 30 degrees
   D. 45 degrees

8. The test used to diagnose whooping cough and pneumonia is:
   A. creatinine clearance
   B. nasopharyngeal culture
   C. ova and parasites (O&P)
   D. breath analysis

9. The sweat chloride test is used to diagnose:
   A. cerebral palsy
   B. multiple sclerosis
   C. cystic fibrosis
   D. diabetes mellitus

10. Occult quantities of blood refer to:
    A. large quantities of blood
    B. small quantities of blood
    C. invisible quantities of blood
    D. hemolytic quantities of blood

11. Which of the following is used as an indicator of clearance in how the kidney is able to remove and filter analytes from the body?
    A. creatinine
    B. creatine
    C. hemoglobin
    D. glucose

12. What is the first step performed in the clean-catch midstream urine collection for women?
    A. Hold the skin folds apart with one hand and urinate into the collection container.
    B. After washing her hands, the patient should separate the skin folds around the urinary opening and clean the area.
    C. The woman should urinate into the specially cleaned urine container.
    D. The woman needs to separate the skin folds around the urinary opening and urinate into the specially cleaned urine container.

13. Fecal specimens are sometimes collected in order to detect:
    A. *Haemophilus influenzae*
    B. *Salmonella* species
    C. *Corynebacterium diphtheriae*
    D. *Mycobacterium tuberculosis*

14. In Figure 16.3, the patient is collecting:
    A. a sputum specimen
    B. a throat culture specimen
    C. a wound specimen
    D. a nasopharyngeal culture specimen

FIGURE 16.3

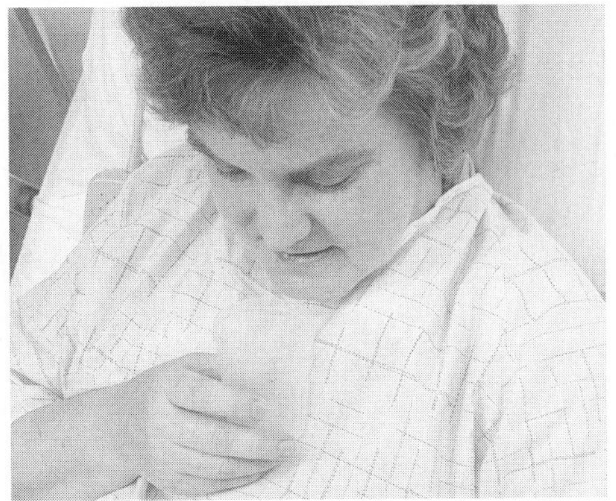

15. What is the specimen of choice for drug abuse testing?
    A. CSF
    B. gastric fluid
    C. peritoneal fluid
    D. urine

16. The presence of bilirubin in the urine may be associated with:
    A. diabetes mellitus
    B. malaria
    C. liver disease
    D. infection in the kidney

17. The sweat chloride test requires the use of which of the following?
    A. EDTA
    B. guaiac
    C. pilocarpine hydrochloric acid
    D. sulfuric acid

18. Fluid from the lungs containing pus is:
    A. seminal fluid
    B. amniotic fluid
    C. sputum
    D. synovial fluid

19. Which of the following is used to detect cystic fibrosis?
    A. breath analysis
    B. sweat chloride test
    C. gastric analysis
    D. O&P

20. Figure 16.4 is illustrating:
    A. the TB skin test
    B. the sweat chloride test
    C. the allergy skin test
    D. the glucose skin puncture test

21. The ColoScreen-ES test is used to detect:
    A. occult blood
    B. hemolytic blood
    C. fungal infections
    D. bacterial infections

22. The second tube of CSF collected through a spinal tap is used for:
    A. clinical chemistry analysis
    B. serological testing
    C. clinical microbiology testing
    D. microscopic analysis

FIGURE 16.4

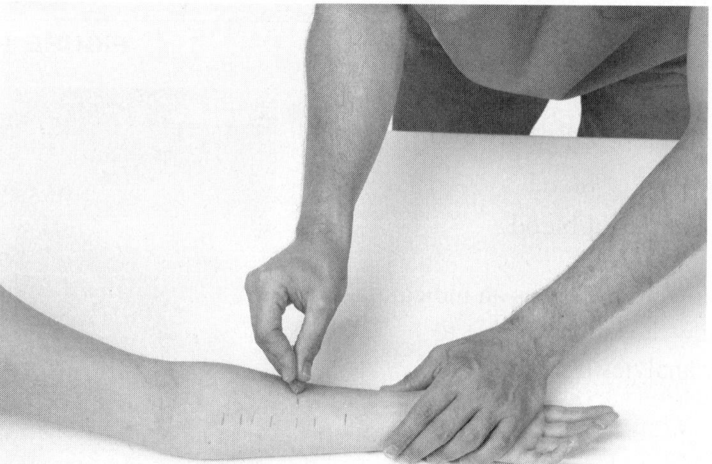

23. What is the name of the disorder of the exocrine glands that affects the lungs, upper respiratory tract, liver, and pancreas?
    A. diabetes mellitus
    B. cystic fibrosis
    C. pneumonia
    D. diabetes insipidus

24. Amniotic fluid can be found:
    A. surrounding the liver, the pancreas, and other parts of the gastrointestinal area
    B. surrounding the heart
    C. around the fetus in the uterus
    D. around the alveolar sacs of the lungs

25. The fluid collected from a joint cavity is:
    A. peritoneal fluid
    B. pleural fluid
    C. abdominal fluid
    D. synovial fluid

26. As shown in Figure 16.5, the patient is collecting a specimen that will be used to diagnose a:
    A. pancreatic infection
    B. respiratory infection
    C. gastric ulcer
    D. hepatic disorder

27. Which of the following types of urine specimens is the cleanest or least-contaminated one?
    A. first morning specimen
    B. timed specimen
    C. midstream specimen
    D. random specimen

28. The O&P analysis is requested on:
    A. CSF specimens
    B. amniotic fluid specimens
    C. fecal specimens
    D. synovial fluid specimens

FIGURE 16.5

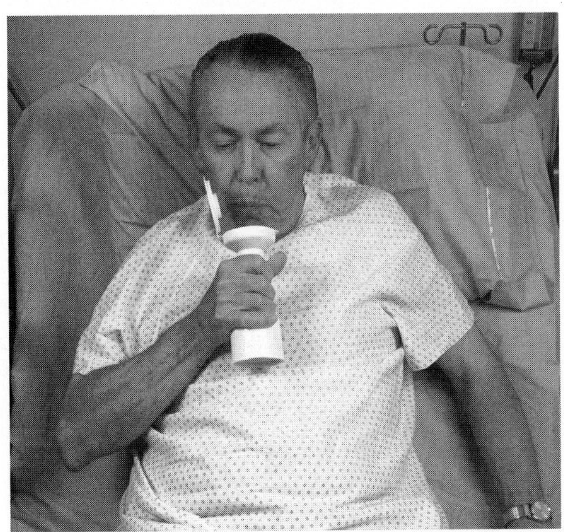

29. For the TB skin test, the diluted antigen should be administered to what part of the patient's body?
    A. dorsal side of the forearm
    B. ventral side of the hand
    C. volar side of the forearm
    D. antecubital crease of the arm

30. A urine C&S should be performed on a:
    A. fasting urine sample
    B. clean-catch midstream sample
    C. 2-hour urine sample
    D. 24-hour urine specimen

31. The occult blood analysis is frequently requested on:
    A. CSF specimens
    B. fecal specimens
    C. throat cultures
    D. seminal fluid specimens

32. BUN test measures the amount of what in the blood and can detect problems with the urinary system?
    A. creatinine
    B. HCG
    C. urea
    D. TSH

33. When instructing the patient to collect a 24-hour urine specimen, what time period is recommended for discontinuation of medications preceding the urine collection?
    A. 4–12 hours
    B. 12–24 hours
    C. 24–36 hours
    D. 48–72 hours

34. A 24-hour urine specimen is usually collected to test for:
    A. hormones
    B. glucose
    C. occult blood
    D. *Neisseria meningitidis*

35. Skin tests are used to determine whether a patient has ever had contact with:
    A. a particular antibody and has produced antigens to that antibody
    B. a particular antigen and has produced antibodies to that antigen
    C. the disease leukemia
    D. the disease polycythemia

36. Which of the following types of specimens is most frequently collected for analysis?
    A. amniotic fluid
    B. urine
    C. CSF
    D. pericardial fluid

37. Fluid composed of products formed in various male reproductive organs is referred to as:
    A. pleural fluid
    B. seminal fluid
    C. synovial fluid
    D. CSF

38. Which of the following can be used in children and infants to diagnose whooping cough?
    A. guaiac smear test
    B. nasopharyngeal culture
    C. O&P test
    D. sweat chloride test

39. When hemoglobin is detected on the urine dipstick from a patient's urine specimen, this indicates:
    A. glycosuria
    B. blood destruction
    C. high chloride levels
    D. leukocytes in the urine

40. The ColoScreen-ES test is run on
    A. synovial fluid
    B. feces
    C. urine
    D. CSF

41. Which of the following is/are included in the physical analysis of a urine sample?
    A. RBCs
    B. hemoglobin
    C. transparency
    D. ketones

42. Throat swab collections are most commonly obtained to determine the presence of:
    A. *Neisseria* infection
    B. *Streptococcus* infection

C. *Staphylococcus* infection
D. *Bacillus* infection

43. Peritoneal fluid is located:
A. around the lungs
B. in the joints
C. in the abdomen
D. in the sac around the heart

44. For the urinary pregnancy test, the preferred urine specimen is a:
A. clean-catch midstream sample
B. 24-hour urine sample
C. random urine sample
D. 2-hour urine collection

45. Ketosis is frequently associated with:
A. liver disease
B. diabetes mellitus
C. chemical poisoning
D. infection

46. Glycosuria is:
A. the presence of glucose in urine
B. the presence of glycogen in urine
C. the presence of glucose in blood
D. the presence of glycogen in CSF

47. Pericardial fluid is collected from:
A. the abdominal cavity
B. the sac around the heart
C. joint cavities
D. alveolar sacs within the lungs

48. Creatinine clearance is determined through the use of:
A. urine specimens
B. pericardial fluid specimens
C. synovial fluid
D. gastric analysis

49. What type of urine specimen is needed to detect an infection?
A. random
B. clean-catch
C. routine
D. 24-hour

50. Nasopharyngeal culture collections may be used to diagnose:
A. whooping cough
B. *Salmonella* infection
C. *Shigella* infection
D. *Crytococcus* infection

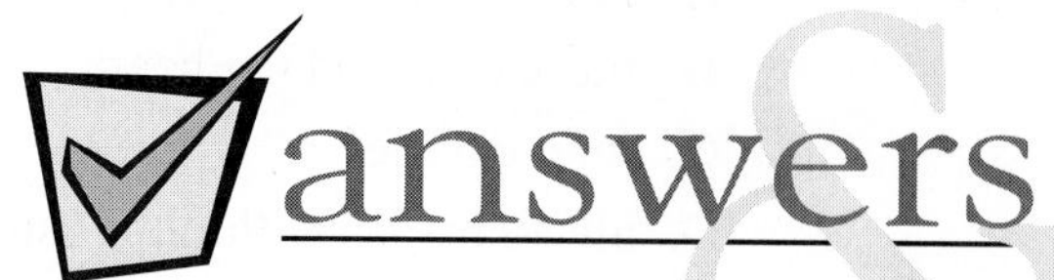

answers & rationales

1.

D. Urine is most concentrated in the morning. (p. 502)

2.

A. Lumbar relates to the spinal vertebrae and thus cerebrospinal fluid is the fluid that is collected through a lumbar puncture. (p. 509)

3.

B. As shown in Figure 16.1, protein in the urine can be measured using the procedure illustrated in the figure. (p. 503)

4.

B. As shown in Figure 16-2, the patient is undergoing a gastric analysis. (p. 517)

5.

B. *Helicobacter pylori* is the bacterium that causes peptic ulcer and can be detected through breath analysis. (p. 518)

6.

A. Glucose level determinations for diabetes mellitus testing should occur on a fasting urine specimen. (p. 502)

7.

B. For the TB skin test, the tuberculin syringe should be held at an angle of 15 degrees for administration of the antigen. (p. 516)

8.

B. The test used to diagnose whooping cough and pneumonia is a nasopharyngeal culture. (p. 511)

9.

C. The sweat chloride test is used in the diagnosis of cystic fibrosis. Cystic fibrosis is a disorder of the exocrine glands. (p. 518)

10.

C. Occult quantities of blood refer to invisible quantities of blood that may occur in fecal specimens. (p. 509)

11.

A. The creatinine clearance test is used to determine the ability of the kidney to remove creatinine from the blood and thus provides information on the kidney's ability to filter analytes from the body. (p. 502)

12.

B. The first step performed in the clean-catch midstream urine collection for women is "After washing her hands, the patient should separate the skin folds around the urinary opening and clean the area." (p. 505)

13.

B. Fecal specimens are sometimes collected in order to detect *Salmonella* species. (p. 509)

14.

A. In Figure 16.3, the patient is collecting a sputum specimen (fluid from the lungs containing pus). (p. 511)

15.

D. Urine is the specimen of choice for drug abuse testing. The end product metabolites of drugs, as well as the drugs, are excreted in the urine. (p. 502)

16.

C. The presence of bilirubin in the urine may be associated with liver disease and obstructive jaundice. (p. 502)

17.

C. The sweat chloride test requires the use of pilocarpine hydrochloric acid. (p. 518)

18.

C. Fluid from the lungs containing pus is sputum. (p. 511)

19.

B. The sweat chloride test is used in the diagnosis of cystic fibrosis. (p. 518)

20.

C. Figure 16.4 is illustrating the performance of the allergy skin test. (p. 516)

21.

A. The ColoScreen-ES test is used to detect occult blood in feces. (pp. 509–510)

22.

C. The second tube of CSF collected through a spinal tap is used for clinical microbiology testing. (p. 509)

23.

B. Cystic fibrosis is a disorder of the exocrine gland that affects the lungs, upper respiratory tract, liver, and pancreas. (p. 518)

24.

C. Amniotic fluid surrounds the fetus in the uterus. (p. 510)

25.

D. The fluid collected from a joint cavity is synovial fluid. (p. 510)

26.

B. As shown in Figure 16.5, the patient is collecting a specimen that will be used to diagnose a respiratory infection. (p. 512)

27.

C. The midstream, or clean-catch, specimen is the cleanest or least-contaminated urine specimen. (pp. 504–505)

28.

C. Stool (fecal) specimens are commonly collected to detect parasites, such as ova and parasites (O&P), enteric disease organisms, and viruses. (p. 509)

29.

C. For the TB skin test, the diluted antigen should be administered to the volar (palm side) surface of the patient's forearm. (p. 516)

30.

B. A urine culture and sensitivity (C&S) test requires a clean-catch midstream urine collection to avoid contamination. (p. 504)

31.

B. Laboratory determination of occult (invisible) blood in feces can assist in the confirmation of the presence of blood in black stools and be helpful in detecting gastrointestinal tract lesions and colorectal cancer. (p. 509)

32.

C. BUN (Blood Urea Nitrogen) measures urea in the blood and is a procedure to determine how well the urinary system is functioning. (p. 502)

33.

D. When instructing the patient for the collection of a 24-hour urine specimen, if possible, the patient should discontinue medications for 48 to 72 hours preceding the urine collection as a precaution against interference in the laboratory assays. (p. 508)

34.

A. A 24-hour urine specimen is usually collected to test for hormone studies or the creatinine clearance. (p. 504)

35.

B. Skin tests are used to determine whether a patient has ever had contact with a particular antigen and has produced antibodies to that antigen. (p. 516)

36.

B. Routine urinalysis is one of the most frequently requested laboratory procedures because it can provide a useful indication of body health. (p. 501)

37.

B. Seminal fluid is composed of products formed in various male reproductive organs. (p. 510)

38.

B. A nasopharyngeal culture is often performed to detect carrier states of bacteria such as *Haemophilus influenzae* and *Staphylococcus aureus.* In children and infants, this type of culture can be used to diagnose whooping cough, croup, and pneumonia. (p. 511)

39.

B. When hemoglobin is detected on the urine dipstick from a patient's urine specimen, this indicates blood destruction with release of free hemoglobin. (p. 502)

40.

B. The Colo-Screen ES test is performed on stool (feces) specimens. (pp. 509–510)

41.

C. The transparency versus cloudiness is detected through the physical analysis of a urine sample. (p. 501)

42.

B. Throat swab collections are most commonly obtained to determine the presence of a streptococcal infection. (p. 513)

43.

C. Peritoneal fluid is located in the abdomen. (p. 510)

44.

C. A random urine sample is the specimen of choice for a urinary pregnancy test. (pp. 502)

45.

B. Ketosis (presence of ketone bodies in urine) is frequently detected in patients who have diabetes mellitus. (p. 502)

46.

A. Glycosuria is the presence of glucose in urine. (p. 502)

47.

B. Pericardial fluid is collected from the sac around the heart. (p. 510)

48.

A. The creatinine clearance test used to determine kidney damage is based on the results from urine and blood specimens. (p. 502)

49.

B. The clean-catch urine specimen is used to detect the presence or absence of infecting organisms. Therefore, the specimen is collected in such a manner as to avoid contamination by bacteria on the external genital areas. (p. 504)

50.

A. Nasopharyngeal culture collections may be used to diagnose whooping cough. (p. 511)

CHAPTER

17 Forensic Toxicology, Workplace Testing, Sports Medicine, and Related Areas

chapter objectives

Upon completion of Chapter 17, the learner is responsible for the following:

1. Define toxicology and forensic toxicology.
2. Give five examples of specimens that can be used for forensic analysis.
3. Describe the role of the health care worker when working with forensic specimens.
4. Describe the role of the health care worker or "collector," in federal drug-testing programs.
5. Describe the function of a chain of custody, and the Custody and Control Form.
6. Give examples of situations where drug testing might be valuable.
7. Describe how to detect adulteration of urine specimens.
8. List two examples of how blood alcohol content is measured.
9. Describe at least three factors that affect testing for alcohol content.

DIRECTIONS Each of the questions or incomplete statements below is followed by four suggested answers or completions. Select one answer that is best in each case.

1. Illicit drugs include:
   A. alcohol and cigarettes for teens
   B. beer and wine
   C. opiates, cocaine, and amphetamines
   D. all of the above

2. Which drugs are the most commonly used by young adolescents aged 12–13?
   A. marijuana
   B. alcohol and tobacco
   C. prescription drugs taken for nonmedical uses
   D. tranquilizers

3. Among drug users aged 14 or 15, what is the most commonly used illicit drug?
   A. alcohol
   B. marijuana
   C. cocaine and heroin
   D. inhalants

4. Gateway drugs are:
   A. cocaine and opiates
   B. amphetamines
   C. inhalants
   D. alcohol and tobacco

5. Addiction is defined as:
   A. drug overdose
   B. a compulsive use of a substance even when it is harmful
   C. heart attack caused by amphetamines
   D. violent bodily reactions to a drug

6. In all 50 states, it is illegal to drive a vehicle while under the influence of:
   A. radiation therapy
   B. steroids
   C. alcohol and/or drugs
   D. pain relievers such as aspirin

7. Which of the following statements defines toxicology?
   A. study and detection of poisons in the body
   B. the study of poisons in urine
   C. legal term meaning illicit drugs
   D. type of specimen that contains toxins

8. Forensic specimens are best described by which of the following statements?
   A. urine or blood specimens that are chemically treated
   B. specimens needed to evaluate liver and kidney functions
   C. tissue specimens from a biopsy sample
   D. specimens evaluated for civil or criminal legal cases

9. Qualitative tests are used:
   A. for screening tests that give a positive or negative result
   B. for specific measures or concentrations of a substance
   C. on biopsy specimens
   D. for forensic specimens that have deteriorated

10. Quantitative tests are used:
    A. for screening tests
    B. for specific measures or concentrations of a substance
    C. on biopsy specimens
    D. only for forensic specimens that have deteriorated

11. A chain-of-custody form, like the one required by the Federal Drug Testing Guidelines, must be completed correctly in order to ensure:
    A. a tamper-evident seal
    B. integrity of the specimen from collection to test reporting
    C. a qualitative result
    D. donor instructions

12. After a specimen reaches its destination, the chain-of-custody process requires that:
    A. an armed guard be on the premises during testing phases and sign-in as a witness
    B. the specimen is never opened to violate the tamper-evident seal
    C. the specimen handler must sign and complete the chain-of-custody form
    D. the donor of the specimen be present

13. The listed acronyms indicate a federal agency and a document that is important to drug testing for federal employees. Which one of the following are the correct names for DOT and CCF?
    A. Department of Transportation and the Custody and Control Form
    B. Department of Toxicology and the Center for Criminal Forensics
    C. Department of Transportation and the Center for Custody Forms
    D. Division of Testing and the Custody and Control Form

14. Professional sports associations such as the National Basketball Association (NBA) and the National Football League (NFL) are among the organizations that have adopted drug-screening programs for their employees. Which of the following statements is *not* accurate in relation to drug-testing employees in these organizations?
    A. Employees have no rights to privacy.
    B. Procedures for collection and testing are well defined.
    C. Employees being tested must initial the specimen label or seal it.
    D. Screening is often done without prior notice to the employee.

15. What is blood doping?
    A. serum levels of marijuana
    B. level of marijuana that produces physical or judgmental impairment
    C. use of blood or blood substitutes to improve endurance
    D. use of steroids

16. Which of the following is the organization that performs over 10,000 drug tests annually on its members?
    A. The Joint Commission
    B. NCAA
    C. ASCP
    D. NAACLS

17. For sports drug tests, urine specimens:
    A. are invasive to the donor
    B. have higher concentrations of drug metabolites than blood
    C. are used only to comply with insurance requirements
    D. are most often used for BAC testing after a traffic violation

18. What is indicated when an employee undergoes drug testing "for cause"?
    A. It means that trace amounts of a drug have been identified.
    B. It is part of every pre-employment physical in the country.
    C. It means that the employee showed signs of being impaired or undergoing unsafe work practices.
    D. It means that the employee did not cause the error in question.

19. DNA testing is often used for forensic purposes to:
    A. track criminals released on probation
    B. determine the cause of death
    C. confirm identity
    D. detect drug levels

20. What is a split urine specimen?
    A. when one specimen is discarded and the second is used for testing
    B. when the donor is required to collect two specimens
    C. when the specimen and test results cannot be considered a valid piece of evidence
    D. the original specimen is divided into two containers

21. In drug screening, which step should be taken to prevent the individual being tested from diluting his or her urine specimen with water?
    A. Bluing agents must be added to the toilet bowl accessed by the donor.
    B. Only use cold water (8°C) in the restroom facility where the specimen is collected.
    C. Add a bluing agent to the urine collection cup.
    D. Videotape the individual during the collection process.

22. After a urine sample has been collected for drug testing and the donor gives it to the health care worker, what is the *first* thing the health care worker should do?
    A. Thank the donor for his or her time and escort the donor out.
    B. Read the specimen temperature within 4 minutes.
    C. Check for evidence of drug abuse.
    D. Take fingerprints of the donor.

23. In drug testing, why would a urine specimen temperature need to be taken after collection?
    A. to check for infectious bacteria
    B. because some illicit drugs raise the temperature of urine
    C. to check for evidence of tampering
    D. to check for fever in the donor

24. Under which of the following circumstances might an employee specimen for drug testing be rejected?
    A. The employee is angry about the procedure and threatens to file a lawsuit.
    B. A friend accompanied the employee but waited outside the restroom during the collection.
    C. The seal on the specimen container is missing.
    D. The donor left the country.

25. Which of the following steps can ruin a laboratory result in collecting blood for alcohol levels?
    A. cleansing the site with alcohol
    B. talking with the specimen donor
    C. vein selection on the appropriate arm
    D. labeling the specimen so that it cannot be viewed

26. How does forensic laboratory analysis differ from other types of laboratory testing?
    A. Specimens may be exposed to rain, mud, or mixed with other human tissues.
    B. Specimens always involve illicit drug use.
    C. Specimens must be identified.
    D. Specimens become the property of the federal government.

27. Alcohol intoxication is defined by:
    A. blood alcohol concentration
    B. whether or not the individual can walk straight
    C. urine alcohol levels
    D. how clearly the individual can communicate

28. The legal limit of alcohol adopted by most states is:
    A. 0.05%
    B. 0.08%
    C. 1.00%
    D. 2.0%

29. A common test method used primarily by law enforcement officials to detect alcohol intoxication is:
    A. a metal detector
    B. a hair testing device
    C. a breath testing device
    D. a specific gravity device

30. What specimen is most commonly used for the detection of neonatal drug exposure?
    A. hair
    B. meconium
    C. blood
    D. urine

31. The term "meconium" refers to:
    A. hair of newborn
    B. intestinal discharge of a neonate
    C. dried blood
    D. urine that contains high levels of amphetamines

32. Which drug is most commonly identified in neonatal testing?
    A. marijuana
    B. cocaine
    C. aspirin
    D. codeine

33. The terms "driving under the influence" or "driving while intoxicated" refer to which category of drivers?
    A. all drivers who drink alcohol
    B. drivers under the age of 21 who drink alcohol
    C. drivers who drink only alcohol
    D. drivers impaired by drugs or alcohol

34. If a drug test reveals a positive result on a meconium specimen, what does it mean?
    A. The athlete used drugs within the past 48 hours.
    B. The mother used drugs within the past 8 hours.
    C. The neonate was exposed to drugs months before birth.
    D. The driver used drugs within the past 24 hours.

35. For commercial drivers (trucks, buses, etc.), what is the legal limit for BAC in the United States?
    A. 0.05%
    B. 0.08%
    C. 1.00%
    D. 2.00%

36. The most accurate means of determining BAC is by testing which specimen?
    A. blood
    B. urine
    C. breath
    D. meconium

37. Measurements of BAC using Breathalyzer tests are affected by:
    A. temperature, breathing patterns, and diet
    B. daylight and wind
    C. cocaine usage
    D. height of the individual being tested

38. How many drinks does it take to get to the legal limit?
    A. 1
    B. 2–3
    C. 4–5
    D. There is not a definitive answer.

39. What are sobriety tests?
    A. a means to confirm identity
    B. tests for balance, speech, or pupil enlargement
    C. methods to determine OTC drug concentration
    D. tests for detecting EPO use

For the next four questions, refer to the following case study when considering answers.

A health care worker responsible for specimen collection and processing in a drug screening facility was on duty when two women came in for a required random employee drug test. The women had similar appearances and were possibly sisters or even twins. The health care worker asked for the identification of the woman to be tested. At first, the woman being tested pulled out a copy of her social security card, and later some other documents. After careful scrutiny of her identification records and contact information, the woman was given instructions about collecting the urine specimen and was asked to go alone into the restroom to collect it. After about 4 minutes, she emerged with the specimen. It appeared foamy and turbid on close inspection.

40. What is an acceptable form of identification?
    A. social security card
    B. birth certificate
    C. photo identification card
    D. library card

41. Which clues could cause the health care worker to suspect an adulterated specimen?
    A. foamy, turbid specimen
    B. the accompanying sister
    C. the time it took to collect the specimen
    D. the facial expressions on the women

42. How could the tampering be confirmed?
    A. Ask the donor.
    B. Take the temperature.
    C. Shake it up to see if more bubbles form.
    D. Test it for ketones.

43. How could this situation have been avoided?
    A. It is impossible to avoid such circumstances.
    B. The health care worker should have warned the patient.
    C. The health care worker could ask the sister to observe her.
    D. Remove all possible adulterants from the collection area.

44. Immunoassays are used for:
    A. screening for drugs
    B. quantitative tests by the NCAA

C. detecting interfering substances in drug tests

D. alcohol breath testing

45. Which of the following substances may interfere with a drug screen?

A. ingesting a poppy seed bagel

B. ingesting French fries 2 hours prior to testing

C. weight lifting

D. coffee

46. What is the purpose of postmortem testing?

A. to confirm DNA identity

B. to help determine the cause of death

C. to perform drug screening

D. to aspirate body fluids for research

47. The term "cannabinoids" refers to:

A. opiates

B. marijuana and hashish

C. oxycodone

D. PCP

48. The class of drugs called hallucinogens causes which type of intoxication effects?

A. uncontrolled singing and dancing

B. changes in hair and nail color

C. improved reflexes

D. altered states of perception and feeling

49. An example of a commonly abused inhalant is:

A. chalk dust

B. anabolic steroids

C. glue

D. opiates

50. Which of the following drugs can be applied to and absorbed through the skin?

A. marijuana

B. anabolic steroids

C. methamphetamines

D. opiates

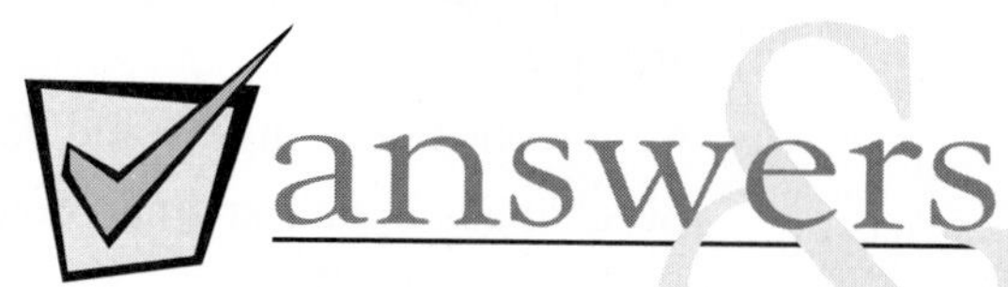

answers & rationales

1.

C. Illicit drugs are illegal drugs such as marijuana (in most states), cocaine, heroin, and hallucinogens. (p. 524)

2.

C. Among adolescents aged 12 or 13, prescription drugs taken for nonmedical uses are most commonly used, followed by inhalants and marijuana. (p. 524)

3.

B. Marijuana is the most frequently used illicit drug by adolescents aged 14 or 15. (p. 524)

4.

D. Alcohol and tobacco are referred to as gateway drugs because substance abuse problems and addictions tend to begin with alcohol and cigarette use. (p. 524)

5.

B. Addiction is the continuing, compulsive use and dependence on a substance despite its negative effects on the user. (p. 524)

6.

C. It is illegal in all 50 states (and most countries) to drive a vehicle (and in some states, a bicycle or boat) while under the influence of alcohol and/or drugs. The drugs need not be illegal and can be the prescription or over-the-counter (OTC) medications. If the person taking the drugs is impaired, they should not be driving. (p. 539)

7.

A. Toxicology is the scientific study of poisons (including drugs), how they are detected, their actions in the human body, and the treatment of the conditions they produce. (p. 530)

8.

D. Forensic specimens are those involved in civil or criminal legal cases. (p. 530)

9.

A. Qualitative tests are often used for screening tests that require only a positive or negative result. Quantitative tests are analytic procedures that measure a specific substance or its concentration in the specimen and produce a definitive amount or level for a test result. (p. 530, 532)

10.

B. Qualitative tests are often used for screening tests that require only a positive or negative result. Quantitative tests are analytic procedures that measure a specific substance or its concentration in the specimen and produce a definitive amount or level for a test result. (pp. 530, 532)

11.

B. A chain-of-custody form, like the Federal Drug Testing CCF, is used to document the handling and storage of specimens from the time of collection to the final disposition of the specimen. (p. 534)

12.

C. The chain of custody is a process for maintaining control of and accountability for each specimen from the time it is collected to the time of disposal. The process identifies each individual who handles/tests the specimen. (p. 532)

13.

A. DOT and CCF refer to the Department of Transportation and the Custody and Control Form. (p. 532)

14.

A. This statement is not accurate. Employees in the NBA and NFL *do have* rights to privacy. Drug test results should be discussed only with authorized individuals. (pp. 534–535)

15.

C. Blood doping is a practice whereby whole blood, packed RBCs, blood substitutes, or drugs are injected intravenously in athletes who try to increase their oxygen carrying capacity and thereby increase their endurance. (p. 538)

16.

B. The National Collegiate Athletic Association (NCAA) tests more than 10,000 student athletes annually for use of banned substances. (p. 538)

17.

B. Urine specimens are used for drug testing in sports because drug metabolites are present in higher concentrations in urine than in blood, large volumes are easily obtainable, there is no pain or discomfort, and it is noninvasive. (p. 539)

18.

C. Employees being tested "for cause" or reasonable suspicion have shown signs of being impaired or have patterns of unsafe work practices. (p. 533)

19.

C. DNA testing is helpful in forensic cases because of its accuracy in identification. (p. 531)

20.

D. A split urine specimen is often used for drug testing. It requires that the original specimen be subdivided into two containers after it has been checked for adulteration. (p. 536)

21.

. Bluing agents or coloring in the toilet and tank will deter an individual from trying to dilute his urine specimen with water. If he does try it, the color of the urine will be significantly altered. (p. 357)

22.

B. When collecting urine specimens for drug screens, urine temperature should be tested within 4 minutes. (pp. 534, 535)

23.

C. Signs of tampering with a urine specimen for drug screens include: unusual color, presence of foreign objects or material, and temperature that is outside the required range (32–38°C or 90–100°F). (p. 536)

24.

C. A specimen might be rejected for drug testing due to many reasons. These include evidence of tampering with it, for example, if the seal on the specimen container has been broken. (pp. 534, 535)

25.

A. Cleansing the puncture site with alcohol will likely cause blood alcohol levels to be invalid. (p. 540)

26.

A. Forensic specimens may be taken from all types of environments and may be exposed to the elements (rain, mud) or mixed with other human tissues. (p. 530)

27.

A. Alcohol intoxication is defined by the blood alcohol concentration(BAC). (p. 539)

28.

B. In the United States the legal limit for BAC is 0.08%, or 80 mg per 100 mL. (p. 539)

29.

C. The most common device used by law enforcement personnel to test BAC is a Breathalyzer. (p. 540)

30.

D. Urine is the specimen most often used for neonatal drug exposure. (p. 539)

31.

B. Meconium is the first intestinal discharge of a neonate, which is greenish and consists of epithelial cells, mucus, and bile. It is also used for drug analysis. (p. 539)

32.

B. Cocaine is the most commonly identified drug in neonatal drug testing. (p. 539)

33.

D. The terms refer to driving a vehicle while under the influence of alcohol and/or drugs. These drivers can be impaired by any type of drug, legal or illegal, with or without alcohol. (p. 539)

34.

C. Since meconium accumulates in the fetal bowel at about 16 weeks of gestation, a positive result can indicate drug exposure to the neonate months before the birth. (p. 539)

35.

A. For commercial drivers, the legal limit for BAC in the United States is 0.05%. (p. 539)

36.

A. Blood is the most accurate specimen (by venipuncture or finger puncture) on which to determine a blood alcohol concentration (BAC). (pp. 539, 540)

37.

A. Breath tests for BAC are affected by ambient temperature, individual breathing patterns (hyperventilation), diet, and fever. (p. 540)

38.

D. There is not a definitive answer to how many drinks a person must have to reach the legal limit. The alcohol content varies on many physiological differences and tolerance to alcohol. (p. 540)

39.

B. Sobriety tests are performed by law enforcement officers who suspect a driver may be under the influence of drugs and/or alcohol. They can include tests for balance, speech, and pupil enlargement or constriction, and if these tests are not completed satisfactorily the officer may ask to do a Breathalyzer test. (p. 540)

40.

C. Acceptable forms of identification that may be used for drug testing include a photo identification (driver's license, employee badge, or identification issued by a governmental agency). Social security cards, birth certificates, and library cards are not acceptable forms of identification because they do not have a photograph on them. (p. 534)

41.

A. The appearance of a foamy, turbid urine specimen should provide a clue to the health care worker that the specimen may have been tampered with. It is likely that liquid soap was added to the specimen container causing this abnormal appearance. Other factors may have heightened the awareness of the health care worker to find concrete clues of a possible adulterated specimen; however, many individuals feel better having a relative accompany them for medical procedures. In addition, facial expressions are not a reliable indicator for the risk of tampering with specimens. (p. 537)

42.

B. The health care worker could document the appearance of the specimen and take its temperature within 4 minutes. This would likely confirm that the specimen had been adulterated. (p. 537)

43.

D. All possible adulterants should be removed from the area where the specimen is to be collected. (p. 537)

44.

A. Immunoassays are commonly used for screening because of their low cost and rapid turnaround time; however, many substances interfere with these tests. (p. 530)

45.

A. Ingestion of poppy seeds may interfere with drug screening tests because they contain trace amounts of morphine and codeine. (p. 530)

46.

B. The term "postmortem" refers to after death. For forensic and autopsy specimens the testing can help determine the cause of death. (p. 531)

47.

B. The term "cannabinoids" refers to marijuana and hashish. (p. 526)

48.

D. Hallucinogens cause altered states of perception and feeling and sometimes persisting perception disorders such as frequent flashbacks. (p. 527)

49.

C. One example of an inhalant that is abused is glue. (p. 529)

50.

B. Anabolic steroids can be applied to and absorbed through the skin. (p. 529)

D. All possible contaminants should be removed from the area where the specimen is to be collected. (p. [illegible])

B. Immunoassays are commonly used [illegible] because of their low cost and quick turnaround [illegible] [illegible] [illegible] their [illegible] (p. [illegible])

A. Ingestion of poppy seeds may cause [illegible] [illegible] [illegible] because they contain [illegible] amounts of morphine and codeine. (p. [illegible])

D. The term [illegible] refers to [illegible] for forensic and other [illegible] [illegible] the testing [illegible] the [illegible] of [illegible]. (p. [illegible])

B. The term [illegible] [illegible] [illegible] and [illegible]. (p. 326)

D. [illegible] [illegible] [illegible] [illegible] and [illegible] [illegible] [illegible] [illegible] (p. [illegible])

[illegible] example of [illegible] that is [illegible] (p. [illegible])

D. [illegible] can be [illegible] and [illegible] (p. [illegible])

B. There is not a definitive answer in [illegible] [illegible] [illegible] [illegible] to [illegible] the [illegible]. The [illegible] [illegible] [illegible] [illegible] [illegible] differences, and [illegible] is advised. (p. [illegible])

39.

B. [illegible] tests [illegible] [illegible] by [illegible] [illegible] [illegible] [illegible] [illegible] [illegible] [illegible] [illegible] the [illegible] of [illegible] [illegible] [illegible] [illegible] [illegible] [illegible] [illegible] [illegible] [illegible] [illegible] [illegible] [illegible] (p. [illegible])

40.

C. [illegible] form of identification [illegible] [illegible] [illegible] [illegible] [illegible] [illegible] [illegible] [illegible] [illegible] [illegible] [illegible] [illegible] [illegible] [illegible] [illegible] [illegible] [illegible] (p. [illegible])

41.

A. [illegible] [illegible] [illegible] [illegible] [illegible] [illegible] the health care worker [illegible] [illegible] specimen [illegible] have been [illegible] with specimens. (p. [illegible])

42.

B. The health care worker could [illegible] the [illegible] of the specimen and [illegible] [illegible] [illegible] [illegible]. This would likely [illegible] that the specimen had been [illegible]. (p. [illegible])

Index

A

D

E

F

M

N

O

P

Q

R

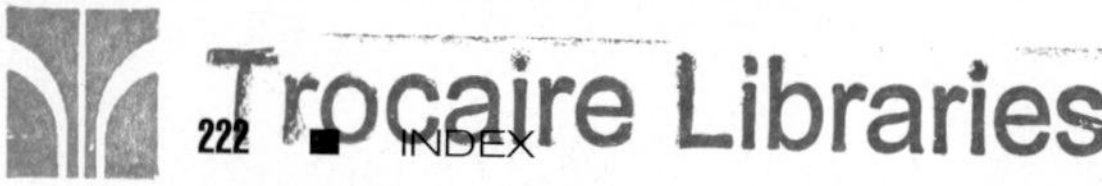